Release

Your Pain

Resolving Repetitive Strain Injuries with Active Release Techniques®

Dr. Brian Abelson, DC
Kamali T. Abelson, BSc

Rowan Tree Books Ltd.
Calgary, Alberta, Canada

Canadian Cataloguing in Publication Data
  Abelson, Brian and Abelson, Kamali

  Release Your Pain - Resolving Repetitive Strain Injuries with Active Release Techniques©
  Includes index and glossary.
  Copyright Registration = 1013747
  ISBN =0-9733848-0-8

Printed in Canada 10 9 8 7 6 5 4 3 2 1

Credits
Cover artwork by Sherry Ward Design
Illustrations compliments of: Active Release Techniques, LLC, Primal Pictures Ltd.
Production and Editing: Kamali Abelson
Proofreading: Hannah MacLeod, Kris Meidal

First Printing: 2003

Kinetic Health books are available at a special discount for bulk purchase by practitioners, corporations, institutions, and other organizations. For details, see our website or contact the Special Sales Manager at Kinetic Health.

Kinetic Health

Web Sites: www.releaseyourbody.com
             www.drabelson.com
             www.activerelease.ca

Canada: **Kinetic Health**
          Edgemont Chiropractic - Soft-tissue Management Systems
          34 Edgedale Drive N.W.
          Calgary, AB, Canada, T3A 2R4
          403-241-3772 (bus) 403-241-3846 (fax)

Table of Contents

Are you looking for effective solutions to your repetitive strain injuries? Then this is the book for you! The following table summarizes the key contents of the chapters in this book.

For a more detailed breakdown, see the following pages for a detailed table of contents.

Table of Contents

Health Disclaimer

This book provides wellness management in an informational and educational manner only, with information that is general in nature and that is not specific to you, the reader. The contents of this book are intended to assist you and other readers in your personal wellness efforts.

Nothing in this book should be construed as personal advice or diagnosis, and must *not* be used in this manner. The information provided about conditions is general in nature. This information does not cover all possible uses, actions, precautions, side-effects, or interactions of medicines, or medical procedures. The information in this book should not be considered as complete and does *not* cover all diseases, ailments, physical conditions, or their treatment.

You should consult with your physician before beginning any exercise, weight loss, or health care program. This book should *not* be used in place of a call or visit to a competent health-care professional. You should consult a health care professional before adopting any of the suggestions in this book or before drawing inferences from it. Any decision regarding treatment and medication for your condition should be made with the advice and consultation of a qualified health care professional. If you have, or suspect you have, a health-care problem, then you should immediately contact a qualified health care professional for treatment.

No Warranties

The authors, publishers, and/or their respective directors, shareholders, officers, employees, agents, trainers, contractors, representatives, successors do not guarantee or warrant the quality, accuracy, completeness, timeliness, appropriateness or suitability of the information in this book, or of any product or services referenced by this book. The information in this book is provided on an "as is" basis and the authors and publishers make no representations or warranties of any kind with respect to this information. This book may contain inaccuracies, typographical errors, or other errors.

Liability Disclaimer

The publishers, authors, and any other parties involved in the creation, production, provision of information, or delivery of this book specifically disclaim any responsibility, and shall not be liable for any damages, claims, injuries, losses, liabilities, costs or obligations including any direct, indirect, special, incidental, or consequential damages (collectively known as "Damages") whatsoever and howsoever caused, arising out of, or in connection with, the use or misuse of the book and the information contained within it, whether such Damages arise in contract, tort, negligence, equity, statute law, or by way of any other legal theory.

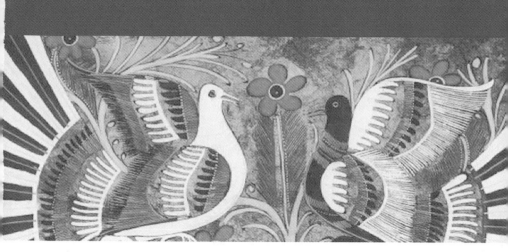

Acknowledgements

This book has taken a tremendous amount of time, effort, and patience to bring to print. And it would never have happened without the support of a great many patients, friends, colleagues, and family. In particular, this book was motivated by the needs of, and questions from, our patients, whose search for more information and understanding of their conditions made me realize the need for a book such as this one.

The first person I would like to thank is my dear wife Kamali (AKA my Indian Goddess). She truly deserves a medal for putting up with me throughout this project. Many times, just as we would finish a chapter in this book, I would decide that whole sections needed to be rewritten and expanded – *for the fifth time!* Besides having remarkable patience, she is an incredibly talented writer who is able to decipher my hieroglyphics and convert them into English; she is my best friend, and my partner for life. Thank you for always supporting me – I could never have done it without you, Babe.

Thanks also go to Dr. P. Michael Leahy, the developer of ART, for his never-ending support and inspiration. Mike is a remarkable individual who I greatly respect as a person, as a teacher, and as the best soft-tissue practitioner that I have ever met. The greatest thing about Mike is that, even though he is surrounded by professional and Olympic athletes, as well as a host of world-renowned celebrities, he is still just Mike. He is humble, easy to talk to, and will always do everything he can to help you. Thanks, Mike, for everything you have done, and for being the inspiration for this book.

I have the privilege of working with some very talented individuals in our clinic. One of these is Dr. Ritchie Mah. Ritchie, besides being an excellent golfer, is also a very talented ART practitioner. By using ART, Ritchie commonly takes the average or professional golfer to the next level of performance. I truly appreciate your sharing your time and your mind as we bounced our many ideas off you!

Next I would like to thank Sherry Sands. Sherry is a very talented Registered Massage Therapist with whom I have the pleasure of working. Sherry has also been a very patient model for many of our photo shoots. Thanks for all your help, Sherry – it is greatly appreciated. Mary Stoddart also needs to be thanked for her help with our exercise protocols. Mary is a very talented Registered Massage Therapist, with a background as a nurse in cardiovascular medicine, and training in Active Release Techniques. Thanks for your help, Mary – you are great.

James Fitzgerald, a fantastic personal trainer and strength coach, worked closely with us to design the exercises in this book. His input and knowledge were crucial as we evolved and tested the best possible exercises for resolving the soft-tissue conditions discussed in this book. James is one of the best personal trainers and strength coaches I have ever met. He graduated from the School of Physical Education and Athletics at Memorial University of Newfoundland with an Honors degree in Physical Education. I have had many professional athletes tell me that James is the best personal trainer they have ever come across in their sporting career. Thank you for everything, James – your help is much appreciated! I also want to take this opportunity to thank you for helping me cross the finish line at the Penticton Canadian Ironman with a swim time, at 46 years of age, that was better than my time when I was 26. Thanks to your coaching, I could even walk the next day!

This book would not be complete without the numerous graphics, photos, and exercise images that make up a large part of its contents. We would like to thank our wonderful models for their time, patience, and participation as we shot, and reshot, the many photos. All of you were great! Thanks also go to Dr. Leahy at Active Release Techniques, and to Primal Pictures Ltd, for their contributions of anatomy diagrams.

A special thanks to Mrs. Josie Smith. Josie is our family friend, office manager, clinical assistant, and the manager of a million other jobs that keep our clinic together. Thanks, Josie, for always being there to listen to my crazy ideas, and for helping us to get this book together! You are the best!

Last, and certainly not least, we would like to offer our heartfelt gratitude to our wonderful proofreaders, Hannah MacLeod, and Kris Meidal. When our eyes were dazed and blurred from the repeated reworking of the text, they helped to find and remove the little (and occasionally big) mistakes that we could no longer see!

It would be impossible for me to mention everyone else that has contributed to this book, with their comments, reviews, requirements, and ideas. To all of you, we would like to take this opportunity to thank you for all your help. This book would not have happened without your support.

Sincerely wishing you the best in health!

Dr. Brian Abelson, DC

About Dr. Brian Abelson

Dr. Brian Abelson is the Clinical Director of Edgemont Chiropractic Soft-tissue Management Systems, in Calgary, Alberta. Dr. Abelson is a native Calgarian who attended the University of Calgary, majoring in Biosciences, before graduating from Palmer College of Chiropractic West, California with an award for *Clinical Excellence*. He holds advanced certification in all levels of Active Release Techniques, is trained in Biomechanics and ART, is an accomplished ART Instructor, and is licensed to the ART Elite Providers Network. He is also the coauthor of the award-winning information websites: www.drabelson.com and www.activerelease.ca.

Dr. Abelson strongly feels that providing a better understanding of soft-tissue injuries, their causes, and the means to their resolution, is a crucial part of reworking our ailing health care system.

In addition to his work with ART, his patients, his teaching, and his writing, Dr. Abelson is a devoted husband, and loving father to two wonderful children. He somehow manages to juggle all his numerous professional activities, his ongoing training as a triathlete, and his family life, while still maintaining a profound joy in life.

About Kamali Abelson

Kamali Abelson is the president of Rowan Tree Books Ltd. She is a Senior Technical Communicator and Information Architect with over 22 years of experience in the fields of science, computing, business analysis, and communication.

She has written, edited, and produced numerous books in fields ranging from engineering, to geophysics, to computing, and health and nutrition. Her published works include online documentation systems, internet sites, user and technical software manuals, engineering manuals, standard operating procedures, whitepapers, and numerous health and nutrition articles.

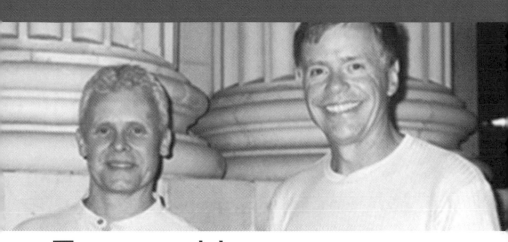

Foreword by

Dr. P. Michael Leahy

ART is a patented, state-of-the-art soft-tissue system that treats problems with muscles, tendons, ligaments, fascia and nerves. Headaches, back pain, carpal tunnel syndrome, shin splints, shoulder pain, sciatica, plantar fasciitis, knee problems, and tennis elbow are just a few of the many conditions that can be resolved quickly and permanently with ART. These conditions all have one important thing in common – they often result from injury to over-used muscles.

Every ART session is actually a combination of examination and treatment. The ART provider uses his or her hands to evaluate the texture, tightness, and movement of muscles, fascia, tendons, ligaments, and nerves. Abnormal tissues are treated by combining precisely directed tension with very specific patient movements.

These treatment protocols – over 500 of them - are unique to ART. They allow providers to identify and correct the specific problems that affect each individual patient. ART is not a cookie-cutter approach. Each course of therapy is individually designed to resolve the patient's problems. Whether you are an office worker, a weekend warrior, or a world-class athlete, the preventative and restorative benefits of ART can help you perform at your best.

Active Release Techniques follows a simple concept, but it is not easy to execute the treatments, nor is it easy to describe how it works. Kamali Abelson and Dr. Brian Abelson manage to describe ART in a way that is easy to grasp - without missing any of the important facts. This is only possible because Brian has a deep understanding of soft-tissue injuries and the methods for treating these injuries. This understanding allows him to make the descriptions simple, clear, and understandable. This is refreshing in a world of overstated claims and hype.

This is *the* book to read for anyone (practitioners, patients, or friends) who wants to achieve an understanding of what causes the majority of soft-tissue injuries, and for anyone who wants to learn how these injuries can be resolved *without* endless treatment. If *you* have a soft-tissue problem, then read this book, and don't be satisfied with anything but the real solution.

Soft-tissue injuries cost more than $200 billion dollars per year in North America alone. With proper treatment, these costs can be reduced to less than one-third of that value. This is the mission of ART; and Dr. Brian Abelson – a certified ART instructor, and an advanced and experienced ART practitioner – is helping us to get there.

Well Done!

Mike Leahy

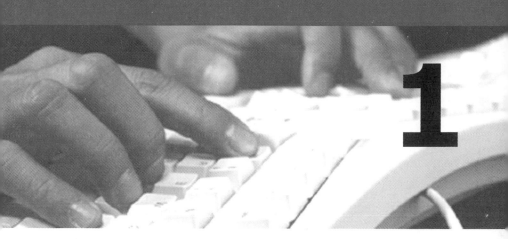

Why is RSI a Problem?

Repetitive Strain Injuries (RSI) have become a major drain on our health care system. RSIs account for over 67% of all occupational injuries, and cost over $110 billion dollars per year in medical costs, lost wages, and productivity.
(*United States Bureau of Labor Statistics, 2001*).

Repetitive Strain Injury (RSI) is caused by repeated physical movements that cause ongoing damage to muscles, ligaments, tendons, nerves, fascia, circulatory structures, and other soft-tissues. RSI sufferers come from many occupations ranging from musicians to meat packers to computer operators.

Repetitive Strain Injury caused by cumulative trauma has become *the* most prevalent cause of injuries in the workforce. RSIs are among the most misunderstood, misdiagnosed, and poorly treated conditions.

Common therapies such as medication, physiotherapy, chiropractic treatment, massage, electrical muscle stimulation, rest, exercise, and surgery have all failed to effectively resolve repetitive strain injuries.

Active Release Techniques® (ART®) provides a means to effectively and rapidly resolve these stressful repetitive strain injuries without surgical intervention, and allows patients to quickly return to their normal activities.

This book will show you *why* these injuries occur, and *how* you can resolve your repetitive strain injuries with treatments of Active Release Techniques combined with effective post-treatment exercises.

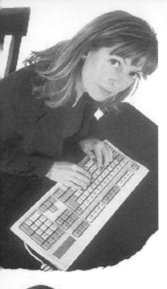

What is a Repetitive Strain Injury?

A repetitive strain injury is a soft-tissue injury in which muscles, nerves, ligaments, fascia, or tendons become irritated and inflamed, usually as a result of cumulative trauma and overuse.

Unlike strains and sprains, which usually result from a *single* incident (called acute trauma), a repetitive strain injury develops *slowly over time*. Other names for these injuries include:

- Cumulative Trauma Disorder (CTD).
- Repetitive Motion Injury (RMI).
- Occupational Overuse Syndrome (OOS).
- Work-related Musculoskeletal Disorder (WMSD).

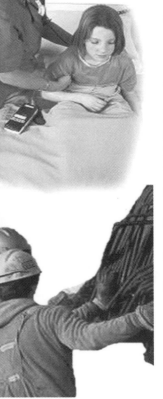

What Causes a Repetitive Strain Injury?

RSIs can occur in any occupation that requires repetitive action and can be caused through the overuse of some part of your body, and by any combination of the following factors:

- Repetitive tasks with many small, rapid movements.
- Insufficient rest time between the repetitive tasks.
- Working in awkward or fixed postures for extended periods of time.
- Excessive and forceful movements, used repetitively, to move loads, or to execute accelerated actions such as lifting, running, hitting, or throwing.

The most common body parts affected by RSI are the fingers, hands, wrists, elbows, arms, shoulders, legs, ankles, feet, knees, back, and neck. Other areas can be affected as well. Computer users make up a large percentage of RSI patients and frequently suffer from repetitive strain injuries to the hand, wrist, arm, shoulder, and neck.

Repetitive Strain Injuries occur as a result of cumulative trauma and overuse of soft-tissues. Soft-tissues that are forced to perform the same job over and over become irritated and then inflamed.

Over time, the cumulative trauma experienced through the overuse of soft-tissues can stress and reduce circulation to these soft-tissues. These stresses create tiny tears in the soft-tissue, which then become inflamed.

The body responds to inflammation by laying down scar tissue in an attempt to stabilize the area. Once this happens, an ongoing cycle begins that worsens the condition. The longer this cycle persists, the harder it becomes to avoid permanent soft-tissue damage. In extreme cases it can cause permanent tissue damage and disability.

How Prevalent is RSI?

Repetitive Strain injuries account for over 67 percent of all occupational injuries.[1] Statistics show that the number of patients suffering from RSI has now surpassed those suffering from back pain. Repetitive Strain Injuries appear in all walks of life, in all types of occupations, and in all types of sports and physical activities.

RSI is particularly prevalent in activities where repetitive, high-force action is required. Nearly two-thirds of all reported occupational illnesses are caused by the exposure of the upper body to repeated traumas.

---

1.   U.S. Department of Labor, Bureau of Labor Statistics, Days away from work highest for Carpal Tunnel syndrome, April 02, 2001, http://www.bls.gov/opub/ted/2001/apr/wk1/art01.htm

Individuals who are at high risk for RSI include those who have occupations that:

- Combine force and repetition of the same motion, for long periods of time, especially in the fingers and hands.
- Require work in awkward or unnatural positions.
- Involve static work positions, while using the hands, arms, and shoulders, or where the torso and neck are held in awkward positions.
- Combine continuous, precise muscular movements with the above-listed factors.[1]

Who suffers from RSI?

Repetitive strain injuries occur in all walks of life including:

- Assembly line workers
- Cashiers
- Computer Operators
- Computer Programmers
- Construction Workers

- Dentists
- Dental Technicians
- Vehicle Operators
- Golfers
- Hairdressers
- Hospital Workers
- Homemakers
- Massage Therapists
- Meat Packers

- Postal Workers
- Poultry Processors
- Nurses
- Tennis and Racquet Sports Players
- Runners
- Triathletes
- Weight Lifters

---

[1]   U.S. Department of Labor, Bureau of Labor Statistics, Days away from work highest for Carpal Tunnel syndrome, April 02, 2001, http://www.bls.gov/opub/ted/2001/apr/wk1/art01.htm

What is the Economic Impact of RSI?

With skyrocketing incidences of RSI, the health care costs for RSI in the U.S. are now surpassing the costs for low back pain as the largest health care expenditure.

According to the *U.S. Bureau of Labor Statistics*, approximately 260,000 carpal tunnel release operations are performed each year, with 47% of these cases considered to be work-related.[1]

Repetitive strain injuries cost over $110 billion dollars per year in medical costs, lost wages, and decreased productivity.

Several years ago, the *U.S. Occupational Safety and Health Administration (OSHA)* predicted that 50% of the workforce would incur repetitive strain injuries during the year 2000.[2]

As staggering as these statistics are, the *National Institute for Occupational Safety and Health (NIOSH)* and a *University of California* study concluded that they likely understated the actual number of cases. They cite that only 44% of work-related injuries are actually reported and the incidence rate may be **130% higher.** [3]

Look at these Statistics!

- In 1981 (when the IBM PC was first released) only 18% of all illnesses reported were RSIs.

- In 1984, RSI cases grew to 28% of all occupational illnesses.

- In 1992, RSI cases grew to 52% of all occupational illnesses.

- In 2000, 70% of all occupational illnesses reported were expected to be due to RSI.

- RSI cases account for one out of every three dollars spent for worker's compensation.

- The average cost of traditional or conventional treatments and disability payments for one injured worker is over $40,000.

This rapid increase in repetitive strain injuries coincides with the increase in the use of personal computers.[4]

1. U.S. Department of Labor, Bureau of Labor Statistics, Days away from work highest for Carpal Tunnel syndrome, April 02, 2001, http://www.bls.gov/opub/ted/2001/apr/wk1/art01.htm

2. U.S. Department of Labor - Occupational Safety & Health Administration, http://www.osha.gov

3. NIOSH - National Institute for Occupational Safety and Health. http://www.cdc.gov/niosh/topics/ergonomics

4. Pascarelli, Emil F., Repetitive Strain Injury: A Computer User's Guide, New York: J Wiley, 1994.

What is the Solution?

In our practice, using a method known as Active Release Techniques (ART), we have successfully treated hundreds of patients who were suffering from RSI conditions.

The *Active Release Techniques - Soft-tissue Management Program*® is forecasted to save employers, health plans, and health care underwriters in the United States and Canada over $100 million dollars in health care expenses, lost productivity costs, impairment claims, and settlements during its first year of operation, and over $1.5 billion within 5 years of the program launch.[1]

We believe that ART is the key to alleviating the suffering caused by RSI conditions, as it addresses:

- The true cause of the problem.
- How to effectively treat the trauma.
- How to stop the condition from returning.

ART has become the solution for many who are dealing with RSI issues today. Read on to find out more about how ART can help you deal with your soft-tissue injuries!

[1.] Statistics compiled by Active Release Techniques LLC.

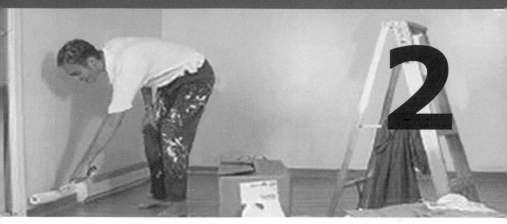

The Specifics of RSI

In this chapter

A serious repetitive strain injury can develop within weeks after symptoms first appear, or it may take years. A repetitive strain injury is characterized by symptoms such as:

- Aching.
- Tenderness.
- Swelling.
- Pain.
- Tingling and numbness.
- Loss of strength.
- Loss of joint movement.
- Decreased coordination.

In general, your injury is more serious if the symptoms:

- Are more intense.
- Are experienced frequently.
- Last longer with each occurrence.

It is important to realize that symptoms:

- May appear in any order and at any stage during the development of a repetitive strain injury.
- *May not* appear during or immediately after the activity that is causing the problem.
- Are not necessarily experienced in the body part where the actual stress is occurring. For instance, if you wake up in the middle of the night with hip pain, that may be a sign of a repetitive strain injury resulting from areas above or below the hips.

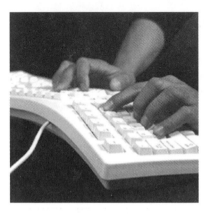

How do RSIs Show Themselves?

Repetitive strain injuries manifest as a broad range of symptoms and conditions. Acute injury and inflammation can result from one or more of the following factors – even without any external forces being applied:

Friction, Pressure, or Tension - Causes an increase in internal pressures and affects already weakened and tight tissues.

Weak and Tight Tissues - Repetitive effort tends to make muscles tighten. A tight muscle tends to weaken; a weak muscle tends to tighten. And on it goes. See *The Cumulative Injury Cycle - page 12* for more details about this process.

Decreased Circulation and Increased Edema - Applies increased forces and pressure upon tissues that are already suffering from decreased circulation. Edema results when pressure is applied over one of the vulnerable, low-pressure lymphatic channels.

External Forces - Constant pressure or a tension injury can also act to decrease circulation and cause further edema.

Adhesion and Fibrosis - Adhesions and fibers are laid down as a result of acute injury, repetitive motion, and constant pressure or tension on soft-tissues.

Cellular hypoxia - Describes a lack of oxygen to soft-tissues that occurs whenever there is restricted circulation. Hypoxia causes fibrosis and results in the formation of adhesions between tissues.

Types of Repetitive Strain Injuries

There are numerous types of Repetitive Strain Injuries, with some of the most common being:

Type of RSI	Symptoms and Variations of Injury
Carpal Tunnel Syndrome (CTS)	Manifests as numbness and tingling of the hand, wrist pain, a pins-and-needles feeling at night, weakness in the grip, and a lack of coordination. See *Carpal Tunnel Syndrome - page 31* for more information.
Achilles Tendonitis	Manifests as inflammation in the tendons of the calf muscle at the point where the tendon attaches to the heel bone. Achilles Tendonitis causes pain and swelling at the back of the leg near the heel, and over the actual Achilles tendon. See *Injuries to the Achilles Tendon - page 109* for more information.
Back and Neck Injuries	Manifests as pain, inflammation, and tenderness to the nerves, tendons, muscles, and other supporting structures of the back. Back and neck injuries include whiplash injuries, disc problems, sciatica, lumbar strains, piriformis syndrome, facet syndrome, and arthritis. See *Back Pain - page 155* for more information.
Elbow Injuries	Manifests as inflammation and pain on the inner and outer portions of the bony prominences known as the medial epicondyle and lateral epicondyle. Initially, it is the tendons that attach the muscles to these areas that become inflamed and injured. Common elbow injuries include Tennis Elbow and Golfer's Elbow. See *Elbow Injuries - page 59* for more information.
Plantar Fasciitis	Manifests as inflammation, localized tenderness, or pain at the plantar fascia, which is a structure that stretches under the sole of the foot and attaches at the heel. See *Plantar Fasciitis - page 95* for more information.
Shoulder Injuries	Common shoulder injuries include Rotator Cuff Syndrome, Frozen Shoulder, Tendonitis, and impingement syndromes. See *Shoulder Injuries - page 73* for more information.

Type of RSI	Symptoms and Variations of Injury
Knee Injuries	Common knee injuries include Runner's Knee, Chondromalacia Patellae, ITB Syndrome, and meniscal and ligament pain. See *Knee Injuries - page 125* for more information.

All of these injuries, and many others, can be successfully and effectively treated with Active Release Techniques (ART). This book discusses many of these conditions, and describes both treatment methods and preventive measures.

The Law of Repetitive Motion

(Copyright: Dr. P. Michael Leahy, DC, CCSP)

Dr. Michael Leahy has defined and tested the *Law of Repetitive Motion*® to describe the physical factors involved in a Repetitive Strain Injury. The *Law of Repetitive Motion* provides a way to predict the possibility of RSI, and also points to possible solutions for addressing RSI problems by altering the key variables.

$$I = \frac{N * F}{A * R}$$

Factor	Description
I	Degree of insult to the tissue as caused by friction or pressure.
N	Number of repetitions of any action.
F	Force or tension of each repetition as a percentage of the maximum strength.
A	Amplitude of each repetition.
R	Relaxation time between repetitions, a time with no pressure or tension on tissue involved.

Your ART Practitioner can help you to manipulate some of these factors to resolve and prevent reoccurrences of RSI conditions. The following image shows a graphical representation of these variables.

Applying the Law of Repetitive Motion

All the following factors must be addressed in order to completely resolve problems caused by repetitive actions. Most of these factors are under *your* control. ART is able to help you to deal with the 'Relaxation' factor. Muscles that are restricted, tight, and adhesed *cannot* relax. By releasing these restrictions, ART can help you to achieve better muscle relaxation, and prevent the return or reoccurrence of the repetitive strain injury.

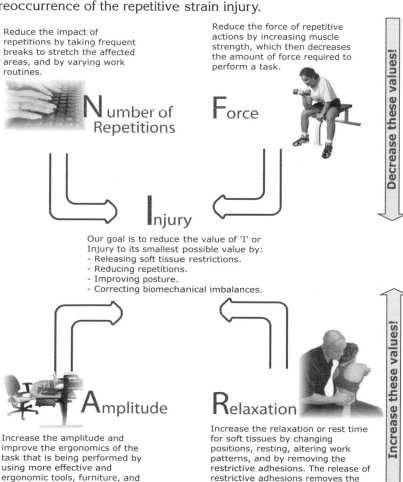

Reduce the impact of repetitions by taking frequent breaks to stretch the affected areas, and by varying work routines.

Number of Repetitions

Reduce the force of repetitive actions by increasing muscle strength, which then decreases the amount of force required to perform a task.

Force

Decrease these values!

Injury

Our goal is to reduce the value of 'I' or Injury to its smallest possible value by:
- Releasing soft tissue restrictions.
- Reducing repetitions.
- Improving posture.
- Correcting biomechanical imbalances.

Amplitude

Increase the amplitude and improve the ergonomics of the task that is being performed by using more effective and ergonomic tools, furniture, and positions.

Relaxation

Increase the relaxation or rest time for soft tissues by changing positions, resting, altering work patterns, and by removing the restrictive adhesions. The release of restrictive adhesions removes the ongoing internal tension and stresses caused by these adhesions.

Increase these values!

If you want more information about how the Law of Repetitive Motion applies to your injuries, read *Applying the Law of Repetitive Motion to CTS - page 43.*

The Cumulative Injury Cycle

The *Cumulative Injury Cycle*® was formulated, tested, published, and copyrighted by Dr. P. Michael Leahy – the developer of Active Release Techniques. This section describes this cycle, and how it applies to all types of RSI.

Note: It is important to have your Doctor first rule out any organic causes of RSI such as arthritis, renal failure, hypothyroidism, diabetes, high blood pressure, and hormonal imbalances.
Most remaining cases of RSI are related to specific physical factors that can be measured and manipulated.

With Repetitive Strain Injuries, the repetitive motion is the cause of chronic irritation to soft-tissue. This irritation creates friction and pressure, which eventually leads to small tears within the soft-tissue. These in turn cause inflammation, decreased circulation, and edema.

Dr. Leahy formulated the *Cumulative Injury Cycle* to describe this escalating pattern of pain, injury, and formation of adhesions.

Cumulative Injury Cycle

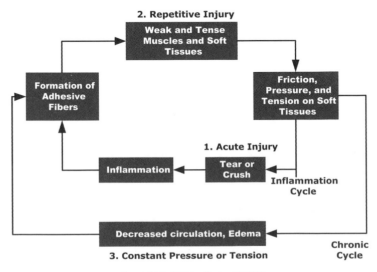

Copyright: Dr. P. Michael Leahy, DC, CCSP

To properly understand the underlying causes of RSI injuries, you must first understand the mechanism and biomechanics of the kinetic chain that created the problem:

1. The constant internal pressure caused by the soft-tissue injury limits circulation to the affected tissues, resulting in decreased delivery of oxygen.

2. Decreased oxygen, or hypoxia, causes several biochemical changes in the body including increased production of mRNA and alpha-1 procollagen.

3. These biochemical changes cause an increase in chemotaxis, proliferation of fibroblasts, and leads to the formation of adhesions and scar tissue.[1]

4. These adhesions and scar tissue in turn create further restrictions, muscle imbalances, inflammation, and swelling.

5. This cycle repeats itself, and escalates in pain, inflammation, and new injuries caused by the restrictive scar tissue.

[1.] Hypoxia-induced VEGF and collagen I expressions are associated with angiogenesis and fibrogenesis in experimental cirrhosis, Christopher Corpechot, Veronique Barbu, Dominique Wendum, Nils Kinnman, Colette Rey, Raoul Poupon, Chantal Housset, Olivier Rosmorduc, Hepatology, Vol 35, No. 5, 2002.

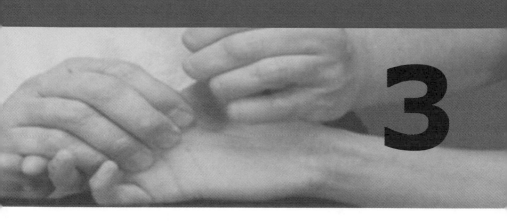

About Active Release Techniques (ART)

Active Release Techniques (ART) is a patented, non-invasive, soft-tissue treatment process that both locates and breaks down the scar tissue and adhesions which cause pain, stiffness, weakness, numbness, and physical dysfunctions associated with Repetitive Strain Injuries. ART is used both for the treatment of RSI injuries, as well as for the improvement of athletic performance.

ART is built upon a strong scientific foundation and is combined with years of practical application in the clinical treatment of soft-tissue injuries. When compared to other medical procedures, ART treatments can reduce the cost of RSI treatment, residual care, and lost productivity to just *one-tenth* of today's normal costs. Even better, ART is able to resolve the true cause of many of these dysfunctions, by providing more than just a symptomatic solution.

What it's Not!

Active Release Techniques (ART) is classified as a multidisciplinary procedure which is practiced by numerous practitioners from a wide range of medical professions and disciplines, including Chiropractors, Physiotherapists, Massage Therapists, Kinesiologists, and Sports Physicians. ART is *not*:

ART is not Massage Therapy! Massage Therapy is able to aid in rehabilitating physical injuries by acting directly upon the muscular, nervous, and circulatory systems. ART and massage therapy work extremely well together as adjunctive therapies, with each serving different functions. Massage therapy, by itself, does not effectively address issues related to scar tissue.

ART is not Physiotherapy! Physiotherapy includes procedures such as manual therapy, therapeutic exercises, and the application of electro-physical modalities. These are valuable procedures, but again, they do not address or resolve the underlying problems caused by the formation of scar tissues.

ART is not Chiropractic Care! Traditional Chiropractic care focuses upon the relationship between the spinal skeletal system and the nervous system; it does *not* focus upon the treatment of soft-tissue. ART and Chiropractic do work well together, but without ART, the results of Chiropractic techniques are often limited in their ability to provide complete resolution for many soft-tissue conditions. Chiropractic works well to release joint capsule restrictions, but these restrictions will return if the original soft-tissue problems are not addressed.

ART is not Surgery! Surgery uses invasive techniques in an attempt to resolve soft-tissue dysfunction. Surgery, though sometimes necessary, often results in numerous physical complications, adverse reactions to medication, and extended time away from work.

As with many other treatment methods, surgery does not address the underlying cause of soft-tissue dysfunctions – the formation and presence of restrictive soft-tissue adhesions that bind soft-tissue layers, and prevent free motion. In fact, surgery usually results in the formation of yet *more* scar tissue. In my opinion, for most cases of RSI, surgery should be the last option to be considered.

ART is not like other soft-tissue or myofascial techniques!

There are many soft-tissue treatment techniques that are currently in vogue, and available to patients today. Many of these claim to achieve results similar to Active Release Techniques, but most are unable to achieve the same remarkable success rates.

Several myofascial techniques use mechanical instruments to perform their procedures. ART procedures do *not* use mechanical instruments, for a very good reason. Over fifty percent of ART procedures and protocols involve the release of entrapped nerves. To *feel* a nerve as it translates or moves through a muscle or other soft-tissue requires a great deal of tactile sensitivity. The process of feeling and locating the relative translation (movement) of a slender nerve fibre through layers of soft-tissue is difficult to achieve with a mechanical instrument.

Adverse reactions to some soft-tissue treatments can include increased inflammation and tissue damage. Excessive damage and inflammation continues the process of adding yet more adhesive scar tissue to the damaged area, and often negates any benefits derived from the initial removal of existing adhesions.

In addition, most soft-tissue techniques only address restrictions at just single points of restriction. Many techniques do not follow the entire length of the soft-tissue structure, nor can they identify restrictions or adhesions at different depths and levels of the tissue. This is in contrast to ART, which aims to return complete translation or relative motion to the full length of the affected soft-tissue and to its adjacent soft-tissue structures. This means complete freedom of motion for the entire restricted structure in relationship to all adjacent structures. Most soft-tissue techniques address only a small aspect of the total restrictions that exist within soft-tissues.

The majority of soft-tissue techniques do not consider the complete kinetic chain in treating a soft-tissue restriction. (The kinetic chain includes all the soft-tissues that are linked to or associated with the affected structure.) Not only do ART practitioners treat the identified area of involvement, they also consider how these restrictions may have altered the biomechanics of the body, and identify and treat the structures that may have been the original cause of the problem.

This far-sighted approach ensures that the soft-tissue injury is truly resolved, and prevents a quick reoccurrence of the condition.

So....What is ART?

Active Release Techniques is a combination of both ART (pun intended) and science. In my opinion, ART provides practitioners with an incredible tool and methodology for effectively addressing the RSI epidemic that is rapidly overtaking our health care system.

As a hands-on technique, ART provides the means for both *diagnosing* and *treating* the underlying causes of cumulative trauma disorders. These disorders often result in symptoms of weakness, numbness, tingling, burning, aching, and numerous other physical dysfunctions.

The goal of ART is to:

- restore optimal tissue texture, tension, and movement.
- restore the strength, flexibility, relative translation, and function of the soft-tissue.
- release any soft-tissue restrictions, entrapped nerves, restricted circulatory structures, or lymphatic restrictions.

ART is based upon a strong understanding of anatomy, physiology, and biomechanics. It is easily supported by science and logic. As a dynamic technique, practitioners are involved in finding new and better ways of improving upon ART's already impressive outcomes.

ART is a true hands-on technique!

ART is a true 'hands-on' treatment and requires a great deal of tactile sensitivity in order to locate, treat, and finally feel the release of soft-tissue restrictions and nerve impingements. During any ART treatment, the practitioner must literally *feel* soft-tissue structures as they translate and glide over and through each other.

ART removes the real cause of the problem!

To effectively treat soft-tissue restrictions, injuries, and chronic pain, ART alters the tissue structures by breaking up the restrictive cross-fiber adhesions (which cause adjacent tissues to stick together) and restores normal function to the soft-tissue areas.

ART protocols allow soft-tissue layers (that were once restricted) to move freely over each other and help to correct a wide range of myofascial and nerve entrapment syndromes.

ART treats more than just muscles!

After years of clinical experience, ART is the *only* soft-tissue technique I have reviewed which effectively addresses the specific translation of not only muscles, ligaments, tendons, and fascia, but also the nerves and circulatory structures that pass through these structures. ART now has well over 500 protocols to address specific soft-tissue dysfunctions. Close to fifty percent of these protocols are dedicated to the resolution of nerve entrapment syndromes.[1]

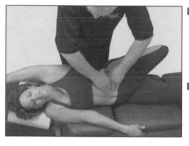

- There are over 200 nerve entrapment sites in the body. When left untreated, these entrapped nerves can lead to numbness, tingling, and loss of function.
- There are several major sites of vascular entrapment. Vascular entrapments that are not released can lead to edema, varicosity, and poor oxygen saturation.

ART is very specific!

ART treatments involve the use of specific treatment protocols that deal directly with the patient's dysfunction. These treatment protocols combine the use of pressure, tension, and motion to force the layers of muscle and tissue to work together properly.

ART has an edge over other procedures as its treatments are very specific and can be customized to each patient's unique needs and problems. Many other soft-tissue techniques use a very limited set of protocols which are then applied generically to all related injuries.

For example, let us look at the *Piriformis Syndrome*, a condition in which the piriformis muscle compresses the sciatic nerve and causes pain in the hip, buttock, and sometimes down through the back of the leg, and into the foot. Most conventional treatment

---

[1].   Active Release Techniques EPN Presentation: *What Does ART Do?* Copyright Dr. P. Michael Leahy.

regimes treat only the piriformis muscle. However, in a syndrome such as this one, it is normal to find that multiple soft-tissue structures are actually involved. When these other structures are not evaluated and treated, the patient ends up receiving a very non-specific diagnosis, inadequate treatments, and correspondingly poor treatment results.

In the case of the Piriformis Syndrome, we normally examine and treat (as necessary) each of the following structures.

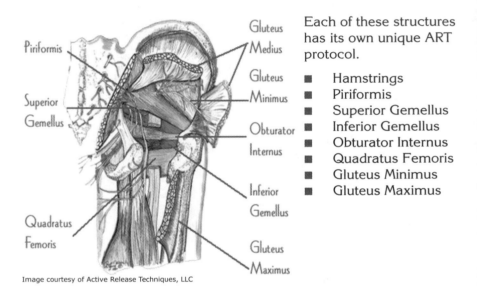

Image courtesy of Active Release Techniques, LLC

Each of these structures has its own unique ART protocol.

- Hamstrings
- Piriformis
- Superior Gemellus
- Inferior Gemellus
- Obturator Internus
- Quadratus Femoris
- Gluteus Minimus
- Gluteus Maximus

ART, due to its touch-based, diagnostic treatment methods, is able to avoid the 'cookbook' or 'recipe' approach to the treatment of non-specific syndromes. Every muscle and every nerve entrapment site is identified, and has a specific protocol and treatment method assigned to it. The 500 specific ART protocols are learned, practiced, and applied by ART practitioners. ART is a dynamic technique; each year, existing protocols are revised and improved, and many new protocols are added to the system. This is in stark contrast to many soft-tissue methods that claim to teach all required techniques within a brief weekend seminar.

To keep ART practitioners at the leading edge of this new information, Dr. Michael Leahy broadcasts weekly clinical review sessions over the internet. These sessions are available to all certified and registered practitioners, and provide the practitioners with direct access to Dr. Leahy for the information regarding the treatment of difficult or unusual cases.

How does an ART Treatment Feel?

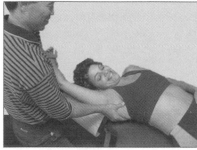

ART is *not* a magic medical bullet or a cure-all. Active Release Techniques *is* non-invasive, very safe, has virtually no side-effects, and has a record of producing excellent results.

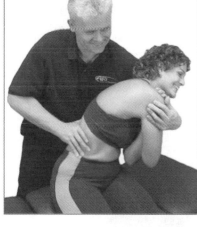

Treatments can feel uncomfortable during the movement phases as the scar tissue or adhesions 'break up'. This discomfort is temporary and subsides almost immediately after the treatment. It is common to feel a duplication of your pain symptoms during the treatment (a good indication that the problem has been identified).

Treatments take about 8-15 minutes for each area treated and may require 6 to 8 visits for optimal results. Patients report that '*It hurts good*'.

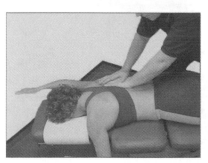

Once a soft-tissue problem has been resolved, the symptoms will not return unless the injury happens again. To avoid future injuries we instruct our patients in specific exercises, give postural recommendations, and explain to our patients the mechanism of injury so that it may be avoided in the future.

Strength, speed and endurance can be expected to improve within the first few treatments. We will often have our patients test these factors after two or three visits. If no improvement is seen, we know that either we have not found the source of the problem, or the affected area needs to be strengthened further.

Why is ART So Successful?

To effectively treat a soft-tissue dysfunction, the practitioner must be able to *feel* the adhesed tissues and restrictions. ART is unique, when compared to other techniques, in that ART practitioners are taught methods for:

- Feeling the location and direction of all restrictions.
- Feeling the breakdown of the adhesed tissues.
- Feeling the change in the soft-tissue as the nerves, tendons, ligaments and muscles translate and move easily across each other.

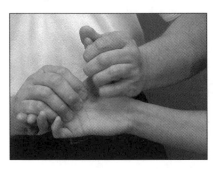

ART requires a strong sense of touch awareness!

ART is used to:

- *Find* the specific tissues that are restricted.
- Physically *work* the soft-tissues back to their normal texture, tension, and length, by using various hand positions and soft-tissue manipulation methods.

This strong sense of *touch awareness* can take a considerable amount of time and experience to develop. ART is successful, where other traditional methods fail, because ART practitioners:

- Locate the true, root cause of the problem. An experienced ART practitioner can successfully resolve many soft-tissue problems within 6 to 8 treatments.
- Locate the restrictive adhesions that have formed, *identify the direction* in which these adhesions are aligned, and *remove* these restrictive adhesions. Compared with ART, most other myofascial techniques are not as specific or as effective.
- Work along the entire kinetic chain. Advanced ART practitioners are also trained in biomechanical analysis and can understand exactly how injuries within the kinetic chain affect the biomechanics of the patient.
- Consider the body to be one complete, dynamic, functional unit – they do not restrict their attention and treatment to just the area of complaint.

Active Release Techniques provides two levels of care – *Injury Care* and *Performance Care.*

About ART Injury Care

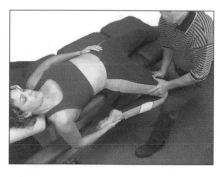

ART Injury Care is used to treat and resolve a broad range of soft-tissue injuries, and return these tissues to full function.

ART Injury Care resolves soft-tissue injuries by removing the adhesions and restrictive tissues that are laid down when the tissue suffers repeated trauma.

Dr. Mah releasing restrictions from the quadriceps.

ART Injury Care removes the cause of the dysfunction, and restores full function, movement, and translation to the affected tissue. ART Injury Care provides the methodology and tools required to return a patient to their chosen occupation, pain-free, and fully functional again. The remainder of this book deals primarily with ART Injury Care.

About ART Performance Care

Once patients have received ART treatments to resolve obvious soft-tissue injuries, they are often keen to return to activities and sports that were previously denied to them by their injury.

At this point, ART can provide patients with a means to *enhance* their sports performance by identifying and releasing restrictions that reduce their performance in that activity. This typically occurs after the practitioner conducts a biomechanical analysis of the patient's motion. During the biomechanical analysis and the subsequent treatment, the practitioner:

■ Evaluates your gait, motion, and posture.
■ Identifies the biomechanical dysfunctions that are restricting your performance.

- Finds the soft-tissue structures that are the primary cause of the biomechanical dysfunction as well as affected structures along the kinetic chain.
- Treats the soft-tissue dysfunctions with ART to restore full function to the affected structures.

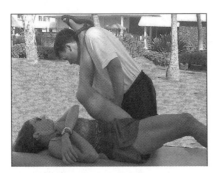

Dr. Abelson at the Kona Ironman Championships - releasing hamstring restrictions.

ART Performance Care is applied *after* trauma-based injuries have been resolved.

ART Performance Care concentrates upon removing those restrictions that inhibit full range of motion, and in restoring full function and performance to those soft-tissues. This process can result in significant increases in sports performance – power, strength, and flexibility.

ART Performance Care has been used to improve athletic performance for everyone from the amateur athlete to Olympic Gold medalists. Many well-known athletes and celebrities have benefited from ART Performance Care, including:

- NHL hockey player – Gary Roberts.
- Figure skaters and Olympic gold medalists – Jamie Sale and David Pelletier.
- Mr. Universe - Milos Sarcev.
- Members of several Olympic teams, including the nations of Canada, United States, New Zealand, and Australia.
- Numerous PGA Golf professionals.

See the Active Release website at *www.activerelease.com* for more details about these and other athletes who have experienced increased performance through ART treatments.

The Bonus...Biomechanical Analysis with ART

Biomechanical analysis of an action or activity is a key part of any ART procedure. ART practitioners conduct a biomechanical analysis of the required action to:

- Determine which structures are affected along the activity's kinetic chain. ART practitioners focus on more than just the chief area of complaint. For example, a runner with a knee injury will often have accompanying restrictions in a multitude of soft-tissue structures above and below the knee.

- Identify the antagonistic structures (opposing muscle groups) to those that have been identified as the primary structures causing the imbalance. Since function and performance is based upon balance and coordination, an opposing soft-tissue structure is *always* affected by restrictions in the primary structure. These muscle imbalances often lead to injuries. Some examples of primary muscles and their antagonists are:
  - biceps and triceps.
  - quadriceps and hamstrings.
  - pectoralis and latissimus dorsi.
  - anterior and posterior deltoids.

ART can help with...

- Arthritis
- Achilles Tendonitis
- Ankle Injuries
- Back Pain/injuries
- Bicipital Tendonitis
- Bunions and Bursitis
- Carpal Tunnel Syndrome
- Compartment Syndrome
- De Quervain's Tenosynovitis
- Dupuytren's Contracture
- Foot Pain and Injury
- Frozen Shoulder or Adhesive Capsulitis
- Gait Imbalances
- Golfer's/Tennis Elbow (Tendonitis)
- Golf Injuries
- Hammer Toes
- Hand Injuries
- Headaches
- Hip Pain
- Iliotibial Band Syndrome
- Impingement Syndromes
- Joint Dysfunctions
- Knee Meniscus Injuries
- Knee and Leg Pain

Once the affected areas (primary structures and their antagonists) have been located, the ART practitioner is able to systematically remove restrictions along the entire kinetic chain. Patients see immediate improvements in their sports performance; from their running and walking speed, to increased power in a golf stroke, to an ability to throw more accurately and at greater speeds or simply with smoother actions.

Who Can Provide ART Treatments?

Proficiency at ART takes a long time to develop. Training is hands-on. The right touch is the most difficult aspect to learn, and takes a strong commitment of time, effort, and resources. This multidisciplinary technique is practiced by Physicians, Chiropractors, Massage Therapists, Kinesiologists, and Sports Medicine practitioners.

ART should only be provided by an ART-certified, soft-tissue specialist, who has been educated in *all* the ART clinical protocols and treatment techniques.

There are many people who claim to practice Active Release Techniques. However, the only individuals who are legally allowed to make this claim are those who have undergone rigorous training and testing with Dr. Michael Leahy. ART practitioners must complete and pass all three sections of ART (Spine, Upper Extremity, and Lower Extremity) in order to receive their certification for Active Release Techniques. To maintain ART accreditation, providers must pass a yearly evaluation in order to receive their recertification in the technique.

Always check the ART website (*www.activerelease.com*) to ensure that your practitioner is currently certified to practice Active Release Techniques, and that he or she is qualified at all three levels of ART. By doing this, you ensure that you are receiving the best and most current treatments.

For a list of ART-certified practitioners in your area, check the official ART website at *www.activerelease.com*.

ART can help with...

- Hyperextension Injuries
- Hyperflexion Injuries
- Muscle Pulls Or Strains
- Muscle Weakness
- Myofasciitis
- Neck Pain
- Nerve Entrapment Syndromes
- Performance Care
- Plantar Fasciitis
- Post-Surgical Restrictions
- Repetitive Strain Injuries
- Rib Pain
- Rotator Cuff Syndrome
- Running Injuries
- Scar Tissue Formation
- Sciatica
- Shin Splints
- Shoulder Pain
- Sports Injuries
- Swimmer's Shoulder
- Tendonitis
- Tennis Elbow
- Thoracic Outlet Syndrome
- Throwing Injuries
- TMJ
- Weight Lifting Injuries
- Whiplash
- Wrist Injuries

The Value of Post-Treatment Exercises

Once the ART practitioner has released the restrictive adhesions between tissues, post-treatment exercises become a critical part of the healing process and act to ensure the RSI does not return.

There are four fundamental areas that must be addressed in any exercise program:

Flexibility - Good flexibility enables muscles and joints to move through their full range of motion. Poor flexibility leads to a higher chance of injury to muscles, tendons, and ligaments. Flexibility is joint-specific; a person may have excellent range of motion at one joint, yet be restricted in another.

Stretching exercises are only effective if they are executed *after* the adhesions within the soft-tissue have been released. Stretching exercises that are applied to adhesed tissues will only stretch the tissues *above* and *below* the restrictions. The actual restricted and adhesed tissues are seldom stretched, leading to further biomechanical imbalances.

Strength - Strengthening exercises are most effective *after* the adhesions within the soft-tissue have been released. Attempts to strengthen already-shortened and contracted muscles only results in further contraction and restriction. This causes the formation of yet more adhesions and restrictive tissues, and exacerbates the Repetitive Injury Cycle (*See page 10 for more details*). This is why the application of generic or non-specific strengthening exercises for RSI seldom works.

Balance and Proprioception - Proprioception describes the body's ability to react appropriately (through balance and touch) to external forces. Proprioception exercises should begin early in the rehabilitation process. Effective proprioception exercises are designed to restore the *kinesthetic awareness* of the patient. These exercises form the basis for the agility, strength, and endurance required for complete rehabilitation.

Cardiovascular - Cardiovascular or aerobic exercises are essential for restoring good circulation and for increasing oxygen delivery to soft-tissues. Lack of oxygen and poor circulation is a primary accelerant of repetitive strain injuries.

The History of ART

Active Release Techniques (ART) was developed, refined, and patented by Dr. P. Michael Leahy, DC, CCSP, a Doctor of Chiropractic, based in Colorado Springs, Colorado, and the founder of Champion Health Clinic.

Dr. Leahy noticed that his patients' symptoms seemed to be related to changes in their soft-tissues. He found that he could feel the changes in soft-tissues when they became restricted or adhesed.

By observing how muscles, fascia, tendons, ligaments, and nerves responded to different types of soft-tissue work, Dr. Leahy was able to develop a treatment system that consistently resolved over 90% of his patients' problems.

Dr. Leahy began developing and documenting Active Release Techniques in 1985 under the initial name of *Myofascial Release*. He used these methods and protocols to treat his patients more effectively and efficiently. Since then, the technique has been patented under the name *Active Release Techniques*, and is widely taught and practiced around the world.

In recent years, Active Release Techniques has expanded at a phenomenal rate. It is taught throughout Canada, the United States, England, and Australia. Practitioners come from around the world to learn and practice this technique. The technique itself continues to evolve and grow as the results of clinical trials are incorporated into the methodology.

About Dr. P. Michael Leahy

Dr. P. Michael Leahy:

- Is a graduate of the United States Air Force Academy and served as a fighter pilot and test pilot.
- Has a background in aeronautical engineering.
- Graduated Summa Cum Laude and Valedictorian of Los Angeles College of Chiropractic in 1984 and became a Certified Chiropractic Sports Physician in 1986.

- Has been proudly serving patients in the Colorado Springs area for over 15 years.
- Teaches ART around the world to practitioners from many different health care disciplines. His efforts have helped to improve the performance of many professional and world-class athletes in sports varying from golf, hockey, football, and weightlifting to multiple Olympic sports.

Aside from helping athletes, Dr. Leahy developed and published *The Law of Repetitive Motion - page 10* and *The Cumulative Injury Cycle - page 12* which have helped to redefine the prevention and treatment of work-related injuries.

More About ART!

So you want more information about ART!

For more details and articles about ART and how it can effectively resolve a broad range of soft-tissue conditions, see our award-winning websites:

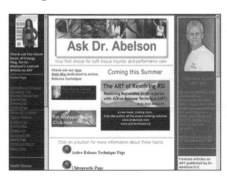

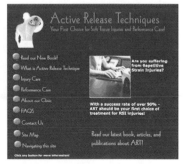

www.drabelson.com   www.activerelease.ca

For more information about ART courses, upcoming insurance coverage, the ART Elite Providers Network, the new ART computer mouse, or answers to other questions about ART, see the official ART websites at www.activerelease.com and *www.zerotensionmouse.com*.

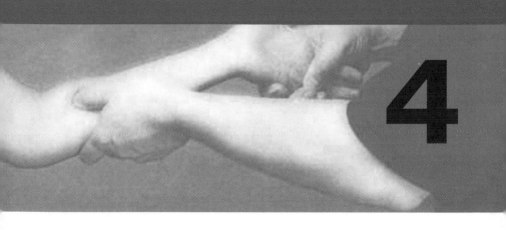

Carpal Tunnel Syndrome

In this chapter

Ask yourself:

- Do you fumble and feel clumsy when lifting objects?
- Do your wrists and hands ache from overuse?
- Do you wake up with your fingers curled and stiff?
- Do your hands burn, tingle, or feel numb?
- Do you drop things easily?
- Do your hands seem to have less than normal strength?
- Do you have difficulty performing tasks such as buttoning a shirt?

If you answered YES to one or more of the above questions, you may have Carpal Tunnel Syndrome or a related Repetitive Strain Injury (RSI). Carpal Tunnel Syndrome (CTS) is the most prevalent, least understood, and most ineffectively-treated neuro-musculoskeletal RSI condition.

What Causes Carpal Tunnel Syndrome

CTS can be caused by any repetitive motion that stresses the upper extremities of the body.

The increased use of computers and their accompanying flat, light-touch keyboards that allow for high-speed typing, have resulted in an epidemic of injuries to the hands, arms, shoulders, and neck. The increased use of pointing devices like the computer mouse and trackball, which require repeated subtle movements, add to these injuries.

The thousands of repeated keystrokes and long periods of clutching and dragging with the mouse causes chronic irritation to soft-tissue (nerves, muscles, ligaments, fascia, and tendons). This irritation creates friction and pressure, which eventually leads to small tears within the soft-tissue. These in turn cause inflammation, decreased circulation, and swelling (edema).

CTS injuries are aggravated by:

- Poor posture and body positions.
- Poor ergonomics (positioning of the chair, mouse, monitor, keyboard, assembly line, and so on).
- Decreased strength due to poor conditioning or injury.
- Insufficient relaxation/rest time away from the stresses that cause the problem.
- Excessive force that is required to perform an action.
- Muscle imbalances.

All these factors place unnecessary, repeated stress upon all the soft-tissues of the neck, shoulders, arms, wrists, and hands.

Who suffers from Carpal Tunnel Syndrome?

CTS injuries occur in all walks of life including:

- Assembly Line Workers
- Bookkeepers
- Cash Register Operators
- Cashiers
- Computer Operators
- Computer Programmers
- Construction Workers
- Dentists
- Dental Technicians
- Vehicle Operators
- Golfers
- Hairdressers
- Hospital Workers
- Librarians
- Meat Packers
- Musicians
- Nurses
- Postal Workers
- Poultry Processors
- Restaurant Workers
- Racquet Sports Players
- Weightlifters

How Prevalent is Carpal Tunnel Syndrome

Estimates about the actual number of CTS cases vary due to poor coordination in the collection and sharing of this information between industry, researchers, and practitioners. However, we do know that this condition is increasing at a phenomenal rate. For example, one study in Canada showed that 614 out of 982 supermarket cashiers reported symptoms of Carpal Tunnel Syndrome.[1]

Over 260,000 carpal tunnel release operations are performed each year, with 47% of these cases reported to be work-related! Additionally, of all the work-related injuries, Carpal Tunnel Syndrome results in the highest number of lost work days. Almost 50% of the CTS cases result in 31 or more days of lost work time! [2]

The costs due to CTS are substantial - both for the patient and for the employer. Consider the costs for a patient with bilateral (both arms) CTS in the United States: [3]

Surgery - Right Hand:	$30,000
Surgery - Left Hand:	$30,000
Secondary Corrective Surgery:	$45,000
Time off Work:	$20,000
Overtime Coverage:	$30,000
Impairment Settlement:	$50,000
TOTAL COST:	**$205,000**

Statistics compiled by Active Release Techniques LLC and presented at the Active Release Techniques EPN Presentation.

1. What is carpal tunnel syndrome?, Canadian Centre for Occupational Health and Safety, March 6, 1998. http://www.ccohs.ca/oshanswers/diseases/carpal.html
2. National Institute for Occupational Safety and Health, CTS Fact Sheet. http://www.cdc.gov/niosh/homepage.html
3. Active Release Techniques EPN Presentation. What Does ART Do? Copyright Dr. P. Michael Leahy.

Traditional Perspectives on CTS

The classical medical definition of Carpal Tunnel Syndrome (CTS) is:

'The impairment of motor and/or sensory function of the median nerve as it traverses through the Carpal Tunnel.'

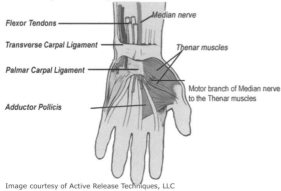

Flexor Tendons

Transverse Carpal Ligament

Palmar Carpal Ligament

Adductor Pollicis

Median nerve

Thenar muscles

Motor branch of Median nerve to the Thenar muscles

Image courtesy of Active Release Techniques, LLC

The carpal tunnel area includes:

■ Nine flexor tendons used for flexing your fingers.

■ The median nerve, which passes from the forearm to the hand through the carpal tunnel passage in the wrist.

■ The carpal bones, which border the carpal tunnel on three sides.

■ The transverse carpal ligament (flexor retinaculum) which borders the carpal tunnel on its palmar surface.

Traditional treatments focus exclusively upon the carpal tunnel, where the median nerve crosses the underside of the wrist, and upon any impingements within that area. These traditional treatments include splinting, anti-inflammatory drugs, cortisone injections, and surgery.

The Problem with Tradition!

Splinting provides temporary relief, especially at night, but over the long term, results in:

• Decreased levels of oxygen reaching tissues. Poor oxygen levels are a primary accelerant of scar tissue creation.

• The formation of increased levels of adhesions between soft-tissues.

• Decreased strength in the arm due to disuse and muscle atrophy.

• Imbalances in body mechanics due to other muscles trying to compensate for the weaker muscles. These imbalances lead to further friction and adhesion formation.

Anti-Inflammatory drugs are useful during the acute stages of the problem. However, several studies have confirmed the fact that NSAIDS (anti-inflammatories):

• Accelerate degenerative processes within the tissues. [1]

• Create drug dependencies.

• Damage the lining of the stomach and intestines.

See **www.rxlist.com** for information about the side-effects caused by your anti-inflammatories.

---

1.   Newman, N.M. and Ling, R.S.M., Acetabular bond destruction related to non-steroidal anti-inflammatory drugs. Lancet, 1985 pp. 11-13.

The Problem - Inaccurate Diagnoses

The median nerve is a peripheral nerve, composed of single cells, which runs the entire length of the arm. This is the nerve that is most commonly associated with carpal tunnel symptoms. Most traditional treatments focus upon the entrapment of the median nerve at the carpal tunnel area.

Research is showing that this traditional emphasis upon the carpal tunnel area is both inaccurate and ignores the greater picture. Dr. Michael Leahy reported that, in over 500 cases of peripheral nerve entrapment, only two cases involved the actual carpal tunnel.[1] In the majority of CTS cases, the nerve entrapments actually occur further up the arm, closer towards the elbow. Our own clinical research has confirmed these findings. Conventional treatments rarely address these other entrapment sites, choosing instead to focus solely upon the carpal tunnel region.

Unfortunately, many practitioners are unaware of this information and continue to use standard medical tests and procedures that focus solely upon the area of the carpal tunnel. Non-specific, inaccurate testing methods often lead to the misdiagnosis (and treatment) of just a *single* entrapment site at the median tunnel, when in fact, nerve entrapments can occur along the entire length of the carpal nerve, from the shoulder to the tips of the fingers.[2] Thus, it is no surprise that most medical procedures achieve very poor results when treating CTS.

The Problem with Tradition!

Cortisone Injections are often prescribed to reduce swelling. Overuse of cortisone causes soft-tissues to thin and weaken, creating a biomechanical imbalance in the kinetic chain. Chronic steroid usage is linked to everything from osteoporosis to immune system dysfunction.

CTS Surgery most commonly involves cutting the transverse carpal ligament at the wrist in an attempt to relieve the impingement on the median nerve and thereby stop the pain.

This technique may provide temporary relief from pain. However, in many cases new scar tissue grows over the carpal tunnel. This scar tissue again restricts the median nerve, resulting in further pain, restrictions, and a reoccurrence of CTS.[3] Patients also experience difficulties opening and closing their hand since an intact ligament is necessary for movement of the thumb and little finger. Remember that invasive procedures, like surgery, should always be the last resort.

---

1. Improved Treatments for Carpal Tunnel and Related Syndromes, P. Michael Leahy, D.C., C.C.S.P. Chiropractic Sports Medicine 9(1):6-9, 1995.
2. The Role of Active Release Manual Therapy for Upper Extremity Overuse Syndromes. A preliminary report. Berit Schiottz-Christensen, Vert Mooney, Shadi Azad, Dan Selstad, Jennifer Gulick, and Mark Bracker.
3. Recurrent carpal tunnel syndrome, epineural fibrous fixation, and traction neuropathy. Hunter JM. Jefferson Medical College, Thomas Jefferson University, Philadelphia, Pennsylvania Hand Clinic. 1991 Aug;7(3):491-504.

Many researchers are warning that such misdiagnoses are a common event. Consider the following typical findings delivered by three commonly used tests.

CTS Test	Test Description	Rethinking the diagnosis
Peripheral Nerve Pain Distribution	Physical examination of a patient diagnosed with CTS usually shows an alteration of sensation in the: ■ Thumb. ■ Index finger. ■ Middle finger. ■ Inner half of the ring finger. The symptoms associated with this peripheral nerve pain are often attributed to impingement of the median nerve at *just* the carpal tunnel.	It is important to remember that the distribution of sensation (or pain) indicates *which* nerve is compressed, not *where* it is compressed. Damage, restriction, or compression in any area of the median nerve makes the entire nerve susceptible to pressure. What initially seems to be a restriction at the carpal tunnel may actually be caused by compression of the nerve in a location further up the arm.
Phalen's Test	With median nerve entrapments, Phalen's Test will cause numbness and tingling in the first three fingers. Phalen's test has been demonstrated to be only 61% sensitive to CTS.	Neither of these tests reveal the actual *location* of the entrapment sites for the median nerve. Many people simply assume that the entrapment is at the carpal tunnel. In addition, statistics show that these tests will *not* identify 27 to 39% of individuals who actually do have some form of CTS caused by median nerve entrapment.[1] Since these tests are non-specific and misleading, practitioners should apply caution when using these tests as a definitive means for diagnosing CTS.
Tinel's Sign	When the median nerve is compressed or damaged, tapping on the Median Nerve will cause pain to shoot down the median nerve. Tinel's sign is only 73% sensitive to CTS.[1]	

1. Tetro, A.M., Evanoff, B.A., Hollstein, S.B. and Gelberman, R.H., 1998, A new provocative test for carpal tunnel syndrome, The Journal of Bone and Joint Surgery, 80 B, 493-498.

CTS Test	Test Description	Rethinking the diagnosis
Nerve Conduction Velocity The not-so-gold standard!	Physical examination of CTS is often confirmed by what is considered to be the gold standard in traditional medicine – the performance of a *Nerve Conduction Velocity Test* (NCV). ■ Nerve conduction velocity testing (NCV) is used to evaluate damage or disease in peripheral nerves. ■ In this test, electrical impulses are sent down the nerves of the arms and legs. The electrical impulse is applied to one end of a nerve. The time it takes to travel to the other end of the nerve is measured. This test only identifies the fact that a specific nerve has a problem. It does *not* show *where* the nerve entrapment sites are located.	Recent research has shown that:[1] ■ NCV studies should not be relied upon to give a "yes-no" answer to the question of whether a person has CTS. ■ People *without* any CTS symptoms are often recorded as having abnormal results on these nerve conduction tests. ■ These tests have been shown to have a poor level of inter-examiner consistency. Again, since these tests can be non-specific and misleading, practitioners should apply caution when using NCV tests for the diagnosis of CTS. The most common misconception is that entrapment only occurs at the carpal tunnel, at the point where the median nerve enters the hand from the wrist.

1. Press Release, The University of Michigan November 9, 1999 Volume 10

The Carpal Tunnel is Rarely the CTS Site

Our own recent clinical experience shows that only **6% of patients** diagnosed with CTS had any significant level of nerve entrapment at the actual carpal tunnel.

For the remaining **94% of the CTS** cases, we found that the most common site of median nerve entrapment actually occurred further up the arm, at the pronator teres muscle. We were able to *resolve* all these remaining cases by releasing sites of entrapment at these other locations. Dr. Michael Leahy, the developer of Active Release Techniques, first reported similar results in 1995. [1]

Thus, it becomes critical that the practitioner examine more than just the entrapment site at the carpal tunnel to properly determine the true location of the median nerve entrapment.

Getting Real Results!

How can you, the patient, determine which treatment method truly delivers the best result? To do this, you need to evaluate the effectiveness of each available CTS treatment method by applying basic scientific analysis:

- Formulate a hypothesis.
- Execute a treatment.
- Review the results.

The correct hypothesis should yield the best results, as defined by the *permanent functional resolution* of the patient's CTS. By this definition, a successful functional resolution of CTS would be:

> '*A patient who returns to full work capacity with little or no discomfort, and who requires little or no maintenance treatment.*'[1]

Remember, a simple removal of pain symptoms is **not** considered to be a successful resolution. You want to be able to return to your job, activities, and your life, with little or no pain and discomfort, and with full function.

---

1. Improved Treatments for Carpal Tunnel and Related Syndromes, P. Michael Leahy, D.C., C.C.S.P. Chiropractic Sports Medicine 9(1):6-9, 1995

The following table compares ART perspectives and results against the perspectives and results obtained by using traditional treatments.

ART Perspectives	Traditional Perspectives
Hypothesis	
CTS is caused by peripheral nerve entrapments at multiple sites, not just at the carpal tunnel. There are many forms of *Pseudo-CTS*.[1] Some of these Pseudo-CTS sites include the: ■ Median nerve at the pronator teres. ■ Radial nerve at the wrist extensors. ■ Ulnar nerve at the medial edge of the triceps. ■ Ulnar nerve at the wrist flexors. ■ Ulnar nerve at the subscapularis. ■ Brachial plexus at the scalenes. ■ Axillary nerve at the quadrangular space. *See page 41 for a picture of these.*	Conventional medicine assumes that CTS is always caused by entrapment of the median nerve at just the carpal tunnel. Most traditional practitioners do not usually look beyond the actual carpal tunnel when testing for and treating CTS.
Treatment	
Using the *functional resolution criterion*, detailed on the previous page, ART treatments show a proven resolution rate of over 90% for CTS. [2] After ART treatments, most patients were able to successfully return to their previous tasks and professions.[2]	Using the *functional resolution criterion*, after surgery, only 23% of all CTS patients were able to return to their previous professions.[3] Some surgeons claim a 90% success rate with CTS. However, many of them are applying a *pain criterion* (removal of symptoms) to their evaluation, rather than a *functional criterion* to arrive at this success rate. Unfortunately, over 36% of all CTS patients need continued and unlimited medical treatment following surgery.[4]

ART Perspectives	Traditional Perspectives
Review	
ART treatments were able to *restore function*, and *remove pain* in over 90% of all treated patients. The vast majority of these patients were able to return to their former occupations with full function, and no pain. This is an extraordinary success rate for this condition. Results such as these have been repeated by ART practitioners' offices across North America.	Over 260,000 surgical procedures are performed each year for CTS. Up to 200,200 of these surgical procedures *fail* each year when the results are reviewed against a *functional* criterion, rather than a *pain-based* criterion.[4] Worse yet, surgical intervention often resulted in further *loss of function*, even when pain was reduced. Patients were not able to return to their former occupations.

1. Overuse syndromes of the upper extremity: Rational and effective treatment. Vert Mooney, M.D. The Journal of Musculoskeletal Medicine, August 1998.
2. Improved Treatments for Carpal Tunnel and Related Syndromes, P. Michael Leahy, D.C., C.C.S.P. Chiropractic Sports Medicine 9(1):6-9, 1995.
3. Bureau of Labor and Statistics and National Institute for Occupational Safety and Health-NIOSH.http://www.cdc.gov/niosh/ergopage.html#epi.
4. Cambridge Scientific Abstracts - Carpal Tunnel Syndrome: An Investigation Into The Pain, Swartz, MA Professional Safety [Prof. Saf.], vol. 43, no. 12, pp. 28-30, Dec 1998.

Why ART is so Successful

Active Release Techniques is successful, where other traditional methods fail, because ART:

■   Locates and removes the true, root cause of the problem – the adhesive restrictions that compress and constrain the median nerve, or other nerves, at multiple locations in the wrist, arm, shoulders, and neck.

■   Recognizes and eliminates the causes of Pseudo-CTS. Pseudo-CTS shows similar signs and symptoms to traditional CTS, but its cause is due to nerve entrapments at locations other than the carpal tunnel, and for other nerves than just the median nerve.

■   Allows the practitioner to diagnose, find, and release multiple peripheral nerve entrapments along the entire kinetic chain – from the hand, to the shoulders, and into the neck.

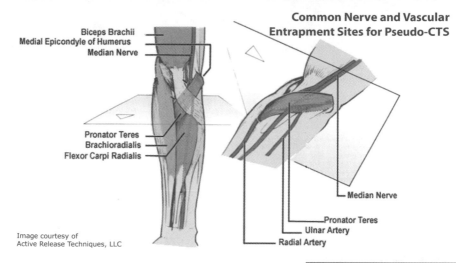

Common Nerve and Vascular Entrapment Sites for Pseudo-CTS

Biceps Brachii
Medial Epicondyle of Humerus
Median Nerve

Pronator Teres
Brachioradialis
Flexor Carpi Radialis

Median Nerve

Pronator Teres
Ulnar Artery
Radial Artery

Image courtesy of
Active Release Techniques, LLC

ART treatments for CTS address all possible nerve and vascular entrapment sites including, but not limited to the:[1]

■ Median nerve at the carpal tunnel and at the pronator teres.

■ Radial nerve at the wrist extensors.

■ Ulnar nerve at the medial edge of the triceps, at the wrist flexors, and at the subscapularis.

■ Brachial plexus at the scalenes.

■ Ulnar and radial arteries at the pronator teres.

■ Axillary nerve at the quadrangular space.

It should be noted that ART treatments for Pseudo-CTS are not restricted to just these sites, but can include other locations in the arm, shoulder, neck, and back.

The actual order and type of ART protocols that are applied varies depending upon the individual, and the exact location of their restricted tissues. ART teaches that the best way to tell if a tissue is restricted in its motion, is by *feeling* that restriction.

Why do Conventional CTS Treatments Fail?

Conventional treatments for CTS often fail since they:

• Usually address median nerve entrapments at just the carpal tunnel area.

• Can exacerbate the condition, rather than correct it, by increasing scar tissue formation.

• Rarely affect the true root cause of the problem – the multiple nerve entrapment sites along the *entire length* of the arm.

• Do not address entrapments of other nerves (radial, ulnar, and axillary nerves) which can also cause CTS-like symptoms and pain. These cases are often diagnosed as standard CTS!

1.   Improved Treatments for Carpal Tunnel and Related Syndromes, P. Michael Leahy, D.C., C.C.S.P.

Other techniques, particularly those using mechanical implements, can never reproduce the sensitivity or accuracy that ART can achieve. Basically, if you can't *feel* the restriction, then you can't *find* it, and you will miss the true cause of the problem.

ART is used to *find* the specific tissues that are restricted, and to physically *work* them back to their normal texture, tension, and length by using various hand positions and soft-tissue manipulation methods. When executed properly, the ART process treats the root cause of the injury by removing the restrictive adhesions that bind soft-tissues, and by allowing free movement of the nerve through the soft-tissues surrounding it. For example, when I perform these ART protocols, I can literally *feel* when the nerve entrapment has been released, and can often feel the nerve itself, as it moves through adjacent structures.

During a typical ART treatment, the practitioner:

- Identifies both the primary and antagonistic muscles that are causing the injury.
- Locates the restrictive adhesions that have formed and the direction in which these adhesions are aligned.
- Determines which other structures are affected along the kinetic chain.
- Uses the hands-on ART protocols to release the restrictions that are the cause of the problem.

Seems simple, doesn't it – and the results speak for themselves. Complete resolution for over 90% of the CTS cases that we have treated with ART!

Splints / Braces

Splints can increase rather than decrease CTS problems since they:

- Restrict motion, increasing stress further up the kinetic chain, which results in yet more restrictions.
- Restrict circulation and the flow of oxygen, causing production of new adhesions.
- Cause soft-tissues to atrophy and weaken.

Weakened tissues force other muscles to work harder, creating a biomechanical imbalance, increasing friction, tension, and the continuation of the Cumulative Injury Cycle.

Surgery:

77% of all carpal tunnel surgeries fail! Even successful surgeries:

- Can result in a permanent reduction of hand strength by 20% to 30%, and cause tired or weak hands.
- Allow only 23% of all CTS patients to return to their previous professions.[1][2].
- Create new adhesive scar tissue which reinforces the original problem by inhibiting the motion of surrounding structures, and creating more imbalances, friction, and pressure.

1.   NIOSH - National Institute for Occupational Safety and Health. http://www.cdc.gov/niosh/topics/ergonomics/
2.   U.S. Department of Labor, Bureau of Labor Statistics, http://www.bls.gov/iif/

Applying the Law of Repetitive Motion to CTS

$$I = \frac{N * F}{A * R}$$

Copyright: Dr. P. Michael Leahy, DC, CCSP

When we look back at the *Law of Repetitive Motion* (*see page 10*), we can soon see that by manipulating each of these variables, we can arrive at a probable solution for CTS.

In this formula, the letter 'I' describes the degree of insult to the tissue as caused by repetitions, force, amplitude, and the lack of rest time. In the following discussion we will show how you, the CTS patient, can manipulate or change the value of each of these variables to resolve your CTS problem.

You need professional help from an ART practitioner for only one of these variables - the letter 'R'. The rest... you can do yourself!

The Letter 'N'

The letter 'N' represents the number of repetitions of any action. Each repetition has a negative effect upon the soft-tissues that carry out that action. You can reduce the impact of these repetitions by:

■ Taking frequent breaks and by varying work routines. Taking frequent breaks does *not* reduce productivity. In fact, several studies have concluded that productivity actually increases with frequent breaks.
For example, a report conducted by NIOSH (National Institute for Occupational Safety and Health) concluded that taking a short break of a few minutes every 20 minutes actually reduced the symptoms of CTS and made workers more productive.[1]

The conclusion is simple! When workers take more breaks they avoid potential problems with CTS, increase their alertness, show greater productivity, and feel increased job satisfaction.

---

1.   Galinsky, T. L., Swanson, N. G., Sauter, S. L., Hurrell, J. J., & Schleifer, L. M. (2000). A field study of supplementary rest breaks for data-entry operators. Ergonomics, 43(5), 622-638.

The Letter 'F'

The letter 'F' represents the force or tension required to perform each task as a percentage of your maximum strength. As you increase the strength of your muscles, you decrease the amount of force required to perform a particular task. If you don't increase your strength, the probability of re-injuring yourself while performing the same repetitive task is very high.

Performing the exercises found at the end of this chapter will help to make you stronger, thereby decreasing the force you need to exert to perform each action.

Remember, there is a difference in the effectiveness of strengthening exercises when they are done before and after ART treatments. Applying strengthening and stretching exercises to an area that is extremely contracted and restricted will only cause an exacerbation of the problem. These same exercises become effective and powerful if they are performed *after* ART has released the restrictions and restored muscle mobility and function.

Making your body strong also makes you healthier! The healthier you are, the faster your body can heal itself. Just consider the benefits that strength training has on your body[1] [2]. Strengthening exercises can help you to:

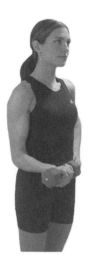

- Increase bone density.
- Speed up gastrointestinal transit time, thereby helping you to digest your food better, and providing your body with more nutrients and energy for the healing process.
- Add lean muscle tissue to your body. Again, the more muscle and strength you have, the less force you need to exert to perform your tasks, and the lower the value of the letter 'F'.
- Increase your resting metabolism, which causes your body to burn fat while you rest, which in turn removes weight-related stress from your body.
- Reduce arthritic discomfort.

1. *Tufts University Diet and Nutrition Letter.* (1994). Never too late to build up your muscle. 12: 6-7 (September).
2. Hurley, B. (1994). Does strength training improve health status? Strength and Conditioning Journal, 16: 7-13.

The Letter 'A'

The letter 'A' represents the amplitude of each repetition. The *smaller* the amplitude, the *greater* the stress upon your soft-tissues. You can modify amplitude by changing the ergonomics of the task you are performing by using more effective and ergonomic tools, furniture, and postures.

For example, the most common cause of Carpal Tunnel Syndrome is the extended period of time spent in front of a computer, using small mouse movements and extensive keyboarding. If you work at a computer workstation, here are some common and effective ergonomic adjustments that you may want to implement to reduce postural stresses, and thereby increase the value of the letter 'A', or amplitude.

Chairs - Ensure that your chair meets the following requirements:

- The bottom cushion of the chair is short enough that you can sit with your back resting fully against the back of the seat.

- The chair has a separate height adjustment, lumbar support, and tilt adjustment features.

- You don't hit the frame of the chair when you push your finger into the foam.

- The chair is not too soft.

Ball Chairs - I often recommend that my patients use a large Swiss Ball or Exercise Ball as a chair for their computer workstation. Ensure the ball is the correct size for your workstation. By sitting on an exercise ball, you are:

- Forced into finding and maintaining a good postural position. The consequence of *not* doing so will result in your falling off the ball! You will find that your body adapts remarkably quickly to keep you balanced and upright on the ball.

- Practicing 'active sitting'. Active sitting requires you to continually adjust and shift your position and balance on the ball to compensate for the other motions of your body. These constant actions help to strengthen all the muscles of your body, increase circulation to your extremities, and improve your sense of balance.

For more information about exercise balls, see *www.fitter1.com.*

Posture - Good posture is a critical factor for increasing the value of 'A', or amplitude. You can do this by:

■ Sitting upright and fully back into your chair. Sit in a manner that maintains the three natural curves of your spine. Adjust the backrest height so that it supports the lower back when you are sitting upright.

■ Adjusting the height of your chair so that your fingers remain in the middle of the keyboard as you move the chair forward.

■ Ensuring your hands and forearms are horizontal and relaxed on the keyboard, and that your wrists are straight with no torque.

■ Ensuring your feet are able to touch the ground. If your feet don't touch the ground, get a footstool.

Computer Monitor - Correct positioning of your computer monitor will help you to maintain a relaxed and correct posture, and to reduce strain and stress on the muscles of your back, neck, and head. You should:

■ Position the computer screen so that the center of the screen is at eye level. The monitor should always be directly in front of you, not off to one side.

■ Position the computer screen to be about 18 to 30 inches from your eyes.

Keyboard - Adjust the keyboard height so that your elbows are close to your body and your arms hang freely. Your elbows should lie vertically under your shoulders.

The Mouse Nemesis - Unfortunately, the standard computer mouse is designed in a way that sets you up for a repetitive strain injury. Normally, when your hand and arm are in a relaxed neutral position, there is a balance between the flexor and extensor muscle of the arm. When using a standard mouse, especially for long periods of time, these muscles become contracted, and remain in a contracted state. This constant state of contraction often results in wrist and elbow problems. With a regular mouse:

■ The extensors tighten in order to hold the fingers slightly above the mouse buttons.

■ The extensors remain continuously under slight tension when the mouse is used for extended periods of time. This causes a repetitive strain injury.

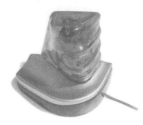

Dr. Michael Leahy has designed a vertical mouse that helps balance these flexors and extensors, and reduce the stress that would otherwise be placed on these tissues by long-term use of a regular mouse. If you are serious about avoiding CTS, I would strongly recommend that you look into this product. See _www.zerotensionmouse.com_ for more details.

The Letter 'R' - Our Key to the Solution!

The letter 'R' for relaxation is the essential key for making the other variables work. The letter 'R' represents the relaxation time between repetitions or the time away from the exerted force. That is, the time with no pressure or tension upon the involved tissue. This is not just external relaxation (such as when you sleep), or the the period of time that you are not performing the repetitive task, but the period of time during which the tissue is not under any type of stress. This _relaxation time_ cannot be achieved with the presence of adhesed or restricted tissues, since the adhesions place an ongoing pressure and tension upon the tissues, and hold them in a contracted state.

It is essential to remove these adhesions in order to allow these soft-tissues to relax and function normally.

ART can be used to remove these adhesions, free up all restrictions, and allow translation and movement of the soft-tissue. By doing this, ART allows the changes made to the other variables to take full effect. Without the removal of the existing restrictions from the soft-tissue, you will find that the changes in ergonomics, force, and amplitude have only a minimal effect.

In Conclusion

In conclusion, you can see that there are many variables that affect and cause repetitive strain injuries like Carpal Tunnel Syndrome. Some variables are easily controlled by changing the ergonomics, strength, and amplitude of your actions; but without the removal of existing restrictions from your soft-tissues, none of these changes will result in long term improvements to your health.

Case Histories and Stories from Patients

Our patients present us with many classic cases that show, over and over, the effectiveness of ART treatments in resolving Carpal Tunnel Syndrome.

A typical example would be Heather. Heather works in a mail sorting plant. For over 30 years, she performed numerous repetitive tasks associated with sorting mail and managing large parcels. She had a perfect employment record until she started to experience problems with her wrist.

The story of Heather's search for a cure started approximately two years before she came to our office.

Heather first started to experience minor wrist pain on the job. Since some of her co-workers were wearing splints, she decided to purchase one to remove some of the stress on her wrist. The splint seemed to help for a short while, but then the pain returned – even more intensely.

Why didn't splints work?

Splints don't work because they:

- Restrict motion, and cause biomechanical imbalances.
- Cause increased stress on other tissues, forcing them to work harder.
- Cause the formation of yet more adhesions and restrictions.
- Slow the healing process by restricting blood flow and oxygen to damaged tissues.

Heather then went to see her doctor, who prescribed some pain killers and anti-inflammatories, and referred her to physiotherapy. These procedures did seem to give her some relief for about two months. After two months, however, the pain once again became unbearable.

At this point her doctor recommended steroid injections which took away all her pain for almost three months. When the pain returned, another series of steroid injections were given. This time, the pain returned within a month.

Heather wanted another series of injections, but her doctor recommended against them.

Why didn't the steroids work?

Steroids and drugs don't work because they:

- Cause soft-tissues to thin and weaken. This stresses the supporting muscles and tissues, forcing them to work harder.
- Reduce swelling on a short-term basis, but do not address the underlying dysfunction – the restrictive adhesions binding the soft-tissue layers.

Heather was then referred to a neurologist, but an appointment was not available for eight months. Heather described these eight months as '*hell days*', during which she was in constant pain. She could no longer work, or perform her normal daily tasks, without feeling excruciating pain.

The Neurologist conducted EMG and nerve conduction studies. The neurologist then confirmed the initial diagnosis of Carpal Tunnel Syndrome (CTS). Surgery was recommended, and a date was set, for *six months later*.

After the surgery, Heather felt great for the first few months. She was out of pain, she could sleep through the night, and she could do her work. However, she did notice that her hands and wrists were very weak. She was told that, in time, her strength would most likely return.

Unfortunately, her strength did *not* return but her **pain** did! Heather then underwent additional physiotherapy sessions, but without any results.

Why didn't surgery help?

When functional criteria are used to measure the success of a surgery, you will often find surgery to be unsuccessful since:

- Hand strength is often reduced by 20% to 30%.

- Most surgeries deal with just the carpal tunnel area.

- Surgeries can create additional scar tissue and adhesions. These adhesive scar tissues inhibit the motion of surrounding structures, and create more imbalances, friction, and pressure.

- Surgeries rarely resolve the root cause of the problem – the formation of the restrictive adhesive tissue.

Several months later, a second surgery was recommended, again after a six month delay. Heather did not see the point in waiting for another six months, only to be disappointed again.

She began to try a plethora of treatment methodologies: Acupuncture, Chiropractic, Massage Therapy, Rolfing, Reflexology, electrical devices, and magnets. Nothing seemed to work, and bills for these therapies were mounting fast.

Heather was desperate when she finally came to our clinic, and the last thing she wanted was to try yet another therapy. Almost the first words that came out her mouth were, "*I don't really want to be here, I know it's not going to work, I am just wasting your time*".

I told her she wasn't wasting her time, and that I enjoyed challenges. She looked as though she wanted to hit me, then started to cry. The poor woman was at her wit's end about what to do.

When I examined her, she showed all the classic pain patterns for CTS. All her orthopedic and neurological tests showed positive for Carpal Tunnel Syndrome. The weakness in her hand was particularly noticeable. She was barely able to squeeze my hand.

Fortunately for Heather, I didn't limit my examination to just her chief area of complaint - her wrists. As I started to palpate further up her arm, I found two very severe restrictions in her *pronator teres* and *scalene* muscles.

- The pronator teres is located in the forearm. The median nerve passes between the superficial and deep heads of this muscle. The pronator teres is actually the most common muscle involved in CTS. [1]

- The scalenes are located in the neck. When the scalenes become tight or restricted, they put pressure on the brachial plexus (a network of nerves that eventually combine to form all of the nerves in the hands and wrist), duplicating symptoms similar to CTS.

- Interestingly, I found *no* restrictions at the actual carpal tunnel.

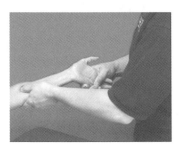

I then proceeded to perform several Active Release procedures on her arm.

Heather was extremely sensitive to any pressure, so the ART procedures felt quite intense as we stripped away the restrictions from her wrist to her neck.

At the end of the first treatment, I asked Heather to squeeze my hand. She said "*Yeah, right.*" I replied, "*Come on, give it a try!*" To her shock and amazement, she found herself able to grip my hand with several times the strength she had shown just a few minutes earlier. Even the pain, which was still present, was greatly reduced.

---

1. Improved Treatments for Carpal Tunnel and Related Syndromes, P. Michael Leahy, D.C., C.C.S.P.

By her 6th ART visit, all of Heather's CTS symptoms and pain were gone, and her strength had returned.

To say the least, Heather was very excited! So excited, that she wanted to share her news with her medical doctor. The doctor's initial response was not very encouraging. He said *"Oh yeah, I sort of heard of that technique, it might help for a while."*

Fortunately, Heather was not satisfied with that lukewarm response. She insisted that he make another appointment for her with the Neurologist, which he did reluctantly.

The Neurologist once again carried out the same nerve conduction and EMG tests. But this time, all the results showed *normal*. Best of all, every criterion that pointed to a requirement for carpal tunnel surgery had also disappeared with the completion of the ART treatments. Heather now had full strength and function returned to her arms and hands, and absolutely no pain. Best of all, Heather has remained pain-free for over one-and-a-half years now!

At this point, it was obvious that Heather had never had any problems at the actual carpal tunnel. Her problems were caused by soft-tissue restrictions further up her arm and neck. Unfortunately, standard tests and methods were insufficient to identify this problem.

I wish I could say that variations of this story are not familiar to me, but they are. The majority of patients who come to our office, suffering from so-called CTS, rarely suffer from a restriction at the actual carpal tunnel. In over 90% of our cases, we can resolve the problem, remove the pain, and restore function by removing restrictions further up the arm, shoulder or neck. Very few cases require work on the area of the actual carpal tunnel.

Exercises for Carpal Tunnel Syndrome

Once the restrictions and adhesed tissues have been released with ART, post-treatment exercises become a critical part of the healing process, and act to ensure the repetitive strain injury does not return. In one study the correct exercises alone reduced the need for CTS surgery from 71% to 43%.[1]

It is important to remember that exercises are only effective if they are executed *after* the adhesions within the soft-tissue have been released by ART treatments.

Attempts to stretch muscles that are currently bound by adhesions often do not achieve the desired results. In addition, only the muscles above and below the restrictions are lengthened. The actual restricted area remains unaffected, causing further muscle imbalances and stress, resulting in the formation of yet more restrictive tissues. This is why generic stretching exercises for CTS seldom work.

In addition to stretching, a program of strengthening is also very important to ensure the problem does not return. The following pages depict some of the specific strengthening and stretching exercises that we recommend at our clinic for the prevention of CTS.

- *Waking up the Nerves - page 53.*

- *Nerve Flossing - page 54.*

- *Golfer's Flexor Stretch - page 55.*

- *Dr. Mah's Scalene Wall Stretch - page 55.*

- *Subscapular Stretch - page 56.*

- *Scalene Stretch with Wall Support - page 57.*

- *Grip Strength - page 57.*

- *Golf Ball Proprioception, Strength, and Endurance - page 58.*

---

1. Rozmaryn LM, Dovelle S, Rothman ER, et al. Nerve and tendon gliding exercises and the conservative management of carpal tunnel syndrome. *J Hand Ther 11*, 1998:171-179.

Waking up the Nerves - This exercise stimulates and wakes up the nerves that extend from your shoulder through to your hand. Do this exercise first, before trying the other exercises in this chapter.

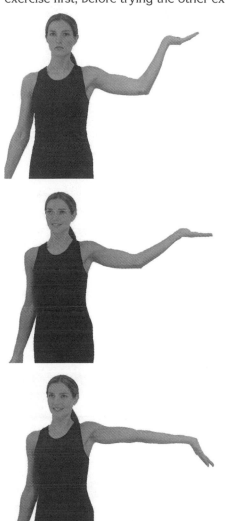

1. Stand in a relaxed posture with the affected arm extended parallel to the floor, with your palm facing up.

2. Bend the elbow so that the forearm extends perpendicular to the arm, and bend your wrist to stretch the fingers of your hand away from the body at a right angle.
   - Keep the upper arm parallel to the shoulder.
   - Keep your other shoulder relaxed.

3. Stretch your arm and hand outwards and try to extend the entire arm so that it is parallel to the floor.
   - Keep your fingers extended and stretched through the entire movement.
   - This exercise should be done slowly, with a slight hold when the arm is fully extended.

4. Repeat this exercise 10 to 20 times until the tension becomes less when the arm is extended.

5. Repeat this exercise with the other arm, for the *same* number of repetitions.

Nerve Flossing - This exercise stretches and helps to translate the radial, median, and ulnar nerves across all the soft-tissue structures through which they pass. This exercise is most effective after ART treatments have been performed to remove the restrictive adhesions that inhibit free movement of these structures.

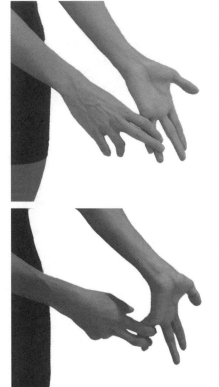

1. Extend the affected arm in front of your body.

2. With the other hand, grasp the ring finger and little finger of the affected hand.

3. With the palm facing away from you, pull those two fingers back towards your body until you feel a strong stretch.

   ■ Hold this stretch for 30 seconds to stretch the ulnar nerve. Release the stretch when you feel the release of the tension in your hand.

4. With the palm facing away from you, grasp the first two fingers and your thumb, and pull them back towards your body until you feel a strong stretch.

5. Very gently, twist slightly towards the thumb for a full stretch.

6. Hold this stretch for 30 seconds to stretch the median and radial nerves. Release the stretch when you feel the release of tension from your hand.

7. Repeat this stretch for the other arm.

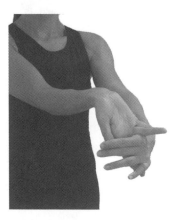

Golfer's Flexor Stretch - This exercise stretches the supinator and extensors of the lower arm.

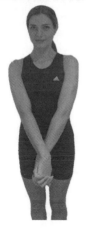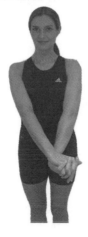

1. Stand, in a relaxed posture, and extend your left arm down in front of you, with your palm facing left, and your thumb pointing down to the ground.

2. Place the right arm over the left arm, and clasp the two hands together.

3. Gently use the right hand to twist the left hand towards the center, until the left palm is facing upwards.

4. Hold this stretch for 30 seconds or until the tension is released.

5. Repeat this stretch for the other hand.

Subscapularis Wall Stretch - This wonderful exercise stretches many of the major muscles of the shoulder and upper arm including the triceps, subscapularis, serratus anterior, teres minor, and teres major.

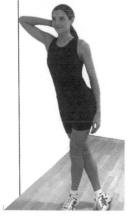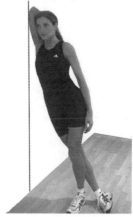

1. Stand about one foot from a wall, with your affected side towards the wall.

2. Place your elbow against the wall and rest your hand behind your head.

3. Take the inner leg and cross it behind the outer leg.

4. Now, lean into the wall so that your upper arm is resting completely against the wall.

5. Hold the stretch for 30 seconds or until the tension is released.

6. Repeat this stretch for the other side.

Subscapular Stretch - This advanced exercise stretches the subscapularis and pectoralis muscles. It requires the use of an exercise ball.

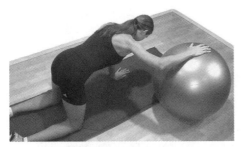

Step 1: Top view - notice shoulder positions.

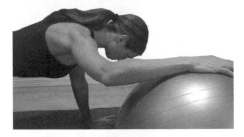

Step 1: Side view - notice shoulder positions.

1. Kneel, with the ball on your affected side, and with your affected arm resting on the ball. Support your weight with the other hand on the floor.

   - Your back, neck, and head should be aligned and straight.
   - Your body should be parallel to the floor with no curvature downwards or upwards.

2. Roll the ball back towards your shoulder until you feel a light tension in the shoulder.

3. Hold this stretch for 30 seconds or until the tension is released.

4. Repeat this stretch for the other arm.

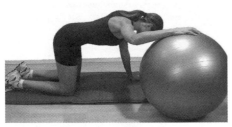

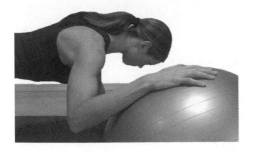

Scalene Stretch with Wall Support - This important exercise stretches the flexors of the forearm, the scalene muscles in the neck, and allows for complete translation of the nerves from the scalene muscles right down to the palm of the hand.

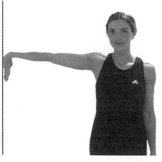

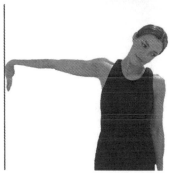

1. Stand by the wall with your affected side towards the wall.

2. Place your hand flat against the wall, with the arm extended, and the fingers pointing downwards.

3. Tilt your head away from the wall and bend your upper body away from the wall. This is a subtle movement.

4. Your head should be tilted as if you were looking at a 'pocket in your shirt'.

5. Hold this stretch for 30 seconds or until the tension is released.

6. Repeat this stretch for the other side.

Grip Strength - This exercise strengthens the muscles of the hand. You will need to use a Power Web as shown in these illustrations. Power Webs can be purchased at _www.fitter1.com_.

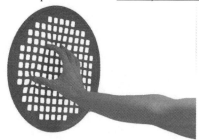
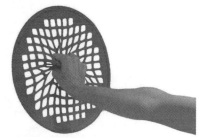

1. Stretch your fingers as far apart as you can and grasp the rubber webbing.

2. Squeeze your fingers together into a fist - without releasing the webbing.

3. Hold the webbing for 5 seconds, then slowly release over 2 seconds.

4. Repeat this exercise 6 times for each hand.

Golf Ball Proprioception, Strength, and Endurance - This
exercise increases your hand's proprioception, coordination, and strength.
You will need two golf balls to do this exercise.

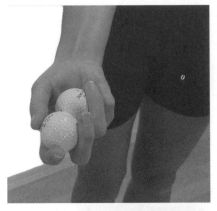

1. With your arm extended, hold the two golf balls in your hand.

2. Using your fingers, rotate the two balls so that they switch positions. Do this for 60 seconds.

3. Now reverse the motion of the balls with the same hand. Do this for 60 seconds.

4. Repeat this exercise for the other hand.

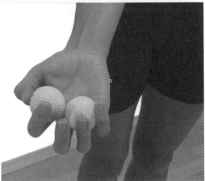

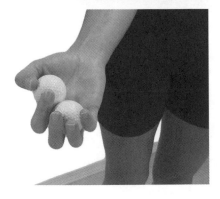

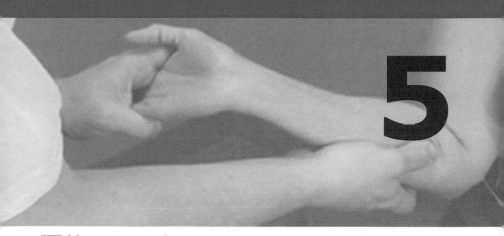

Elbow Injuries

In this chapter

Ask yourself:

- Do you have a burning sensation, tenderness, or pain on the outside or inside of the elbow?

- Do you have pain that spreads from your elbow to your wrist?

- Does your elbow pain get worse when you extend or flex your wrist?

- Does your elbow pain get worse when you grasp objects?

- Do twisting actions of the forearm increase elbow pain?

- Has your ability to extend or flex your elbow decreased?

If you answered YES to one or more of the above questions, you may have an elbow injury. These injuries are commonly diagnosed as Golfer's Elbow, Tennis Elbow, Bursitis, Ulnar Nerve Entrapment, Radial Nerve Entrapment, or Tendonitis.

Active Release Techniques can be used to effectively treat and resolve the majority of these cases within a very short time period.

About the Elbow

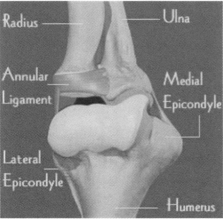

Image courtesy of Primal Pictures Ltd.
www.anatomy.tv

The elbow is a hinge joint which serves as the link between the bones of the upper arm and forearm. This joint consists of three bones (humerus, ulna, and radius).

On the inside of the elbow, the flexor muscles attach to the common flexor tendon which then attaches to the medial epicondyle of the humerus. Flexor muscles run from the medial epicondyle down to the wrist.

On the outside of the elbow, the extensor muscles attach to the common extensor tendon which in turn attaches to the lateral epicondyle of the humerus. Extensor muscles run from the lateral epicondyle down to the wrist.

When the muscles involved in extension and flexion of the elbow are overused, the attachment points at the elbow (the common flexor tendon and the common extensor tendon) become inflamed and very painful.

This causes the body to lay down scar tissue which binds these tendons to the overlaying soft-tissue layers, restricting motion, and preventing the smooth translation of these soft-tissues.

The muscles involved in elbow flexion are:
- Flexor Digitorum Profundus
- Flexor Pollicis Longus
- Flexor Digitorum Superficialis
- Pronator Teres
- Flexor Carpi Radialis
- Palmaris Longus
- Flexor Carpi Ulnaris
- Brachioradialis

The muscles involved in elbow extension are:
- Brachioradialis
- Extensor carpi radialis longus
- Extensor carpi radialis brevis
- Extensor digitorum
- Extensor digiti minimi
- Extensor carpi ulnaris
- Supinator
- Abductor pollicis longus

What Causes Elbow Injuries

Elbow injuries can be caused by:

- Acute trauma.
- Repetitive motions.
- Muscle imbalances.
- Lack of soft-tissue translation or movement.

This chapter focuses on elbow injuries that are caused by repetitive actions and the resulting muscle imbalances caused by these actions.

In most cases of elbow pain, muscles become shortened due to injury, trauma, or from repetitive strains which then cause micro-tears. Usually more than one muscle is involved. To compensate for the stresses placed upon the elbow, the body lays down fibrous adhesions between these muscles.

The scar tissue which forms at the injury site is less elastic, and more fibrotic, than normal tissue, causing muscles to gradually lose their ability to stretch. Shortened tight muscles are weaker and more prone to injury.

These adhesions restrict the muscle's ability to slide freely past one another, they disrupt joint mechanics, and they cause the muscles to feel tight. Shortened muscles and tightened joints all combine to impair coordination and reduce power, resulting in further injuries. This cycle will repeat itself unless these restrictions are released.

Two of the most common repetitive strain elbow injuries are:

- Golfer's Elbow (medial epicondylitis).
- Tennis Elbow (lateral epicondylitis).

Although these injuries occur at different points in the elbow and involve different structures, the basic concepts for treatment and exercise remain similar.

Who suffers from Elbow Injuries?

Elbow injuries that are caused by repetitive actions occur in a broad range of professions, including:

- Baseball Players
- Computer Operators
- Football Players
- Golfers
- Hairdressers
- Inline Skaters
- Keyboard Operators
- Meat Packers
- Musicians
- Postal /Factory Workers
- Nurses
- Racquet Sports Players
- Word Processors

Traditional Treatments for Elbow Injuries

Elbow injuries are traditionally treated with one or more of the following:

- Anti-inflammatories
- Braces
- Cortisone shots
- Cross-fiber massage
- Physiotherapy
- Ultrasound

61

Evaluating Golf Biomechanics

We regularly hold clinics where we evaluate golf swing biomechanics to identify soft-tissue imbalances that affect the strength and accuracy of the golfer's swing.

Common swing faults occur due to tight shoulders, tightness in the hip joint, spinal injuries, and repetitive strain injuries.

For example, when shoulder rotation is restricted the body compensates with excessive spinal rotation. This can result in back injury if, as it is with most people, full flexibility is lacking in the spine. In addition, golfers will notice that they have difficulties in:

- Keeping their eyes on the ball.
- Maintaining an optimal swing plane.

This results in fat or thin shots. When the golfer attempts to compensate at the shoulder joint, the chance of a hook or slice increases. Tightness in the rotational muscles of the hip joint places additional strain on the shoulder and spine as they rotate through the golf swing. Often a golfer will compensate by lifting up during the backswing and then chopping down on the ball, resulting in a fat shot.

A Patient's Story

As a golf pro who is very active in competitive professional golf events, keeping my swing limber and pain-free is extremely important to me.

At age 43, a life of golf and other athletic endeavors has left me with numerous small injuries, tight muscles, and chronic sore back issues.

The help I received from the experts with their ART techniques have truly helped me. I find they can quickly get rid of tight and sore areas that would otherwise limit the range of motion in my golf swing as well as in my everyday life.

Gordon Courage
Canadian PGA Golf Pro

Wrist and elbow injuries often occur when the body does not have the capacity to effectively compensate for restrictions at the shoulder, spine, or hips. The wrists are then over-used to drive, as well as decelerate, the golf club. By correcting soft-tissue imbalances throughout the body, we are often able to prevent injuries such as Golfer's Elbow from occurring, and are able to help the golfer perform better at his or her game.

Note: The concepts and ideas for swing biomechanics are beyond the scope of this book, but will be addressed in our upcoming book about ART Performance Care and Golf Injuries. Stay tuned!

Golfer's Elbow

Golfer's Elbow refers to the pain and inflammation that occurs at the inside point of the elbow (medial epicondylitis).

Golfer's Elbow can be caused by any activity (not just golf) that requires forceful and repeated bending of the wrist and fingers. When the golfer swings his club, the flexor muscles and tendons of the arm tighten just before the club makes contact with the ball.

This repeated action stresses the muscles, causing micro-tearing of the flexor tendon, and inflammation of the soft-tissues. RSI problems occur when these muscles and tendons continue to be re-injured while the small tears are still in the process of healing. These new injuries cause the body to lay down additional adhesive scar tissue between the muscle layers in an attempt to stabilize the affected soft-tissues.

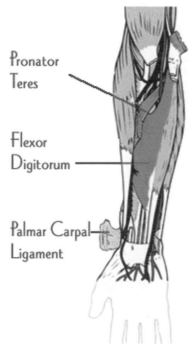

Pronator
Teres

Flexor
Digitorum

Palmar Carpal
Ligament

This adhesive scar tissue forms attachments between adjacent structures and inhibits the normal movement or translation of soft-tissue structures. This lack of smooth movement causes friction and generates an ongoing cycle of inflammation and scar tissue formation. For more information about this process, see *The Cumulative Injury Cycle - page 12.*

In most cases, Active Release Techniques could prevent or greatly reduce this type of injury. See *How ART Corrects Elbow Injuries - page 66* for more details about how ART is used to correct golfers-elbow-related injuries.

Image courtesy of Active Release Techniques, LLC

Tennis Elbow

Tennis Elbow is a painful condition of the outside point of the elbow that typically involves inflammation and irritation of the extensor tendon where it attaches to the lateral epicondyle.

The process of injury for Tennis Elbow (lateral epicondylitis) is identical to that of Golfer's Elbow (medial epicondylitis). However, for Tennis Elbow, the pain manifests on the *outside* point of the elbow.

Tennis Elbow involves the extensors (the muscles that bend the wrist back). The extensors attach to the lateral epicondyle, on the outside of the elbow. The common extensor tendon also attaches to the lateral epicondyle. Both these structures are susceptible to micro-tears when they are exposed to repetitive actions.

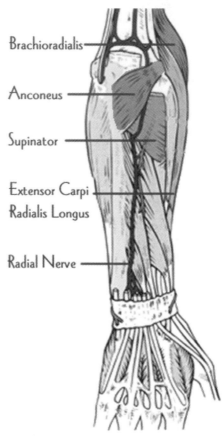

Brachioradialis

Anconeus

Supinator

Extensor Carpi Radialis Longus

Radial Nerve

Image courtesy of
Active Release Techniques, LLC

As with Golfer's Elbow, the so-called Tennis Elbow can be caused by a variety of activities. Any activity that involves supination (turning the hand, palm side up), or lifting objects with your elbow in full extension (elbow straight) can cause this condition.

The repetitive motions of these activities result in micro-tears, inflammation, scar tissue formation, and physical dysfunctions that then manifest as Tennis Elbow. Several layers of soft-tissues are involved in the injury, including:

- The deep annular ligament.
- The supinator and anconeus muscles.
- The superficial structures of the extensor muscles.

In most cases, Active Release Techniques could prevent or greatly reduce this type of injury. See *How ART Corrects Elbow Injuries - page 66* for more details about how ART is used to correct tennis-elbow-related injuries.

Specific ART procedures are used to treat *each layer* of the injury. These ART procedures release the restrictive adhesions that bind these soft-tissue layers together, and allow the tissues to once again move smoothly over each other.

Through touch and practice, the ART practitioner can literally *feel* when this has been achieved. In most cases, the patient experiences an immediate decrease in pain, and an increase in range of motion and strength.

A Patient's Story

I have suffered from Tennis Elbow for over 16 years. I tried all the traditional remedies from physiotherapy to cortisone shots, but nothing worked.

My arm started to go numb and I couldn't even sleep at night any more. My wrist was continually aching and I wore a wrist brace to get through the day. It got to the point where the pain was so bad that I relinquished and had another cortisone shot, and found that didn't work at all.

A friend saw the trouble I was having and mentioned that his son-in-law had received ART treatments and that it had worked wonders for him.

I contacted Dr. Abelson. After an initial treatment, he indicated that just 4 or 5 treatments should have my elbow back in good order.

The difference was amazing after just the first treatment, and with the exercises he prescribed. After just five treatments, my elbow is almost pain free, and is continuously getting better.

Louis Tighe

How ART Corrects Elbow Injuries

For the majority of cases, I consider elbow injuries to be very easy to treat when using Active Release Techniques. In fact, for many years, I had not realized how ineffective other methods were for treating this type of injury. We often hear about how a patient has suffered for years, trying numerous types of therapies, with little or no success.

At our clinic, we are able to resolve most elbow injuries within 6 to 8 visits. Many medical professionals and patients cannot believe that we can achieve results so quickly, especially when the patient has already been through extended therapy prior to visiting us.

In order to effectively balance your muscles and remove joint restrictions we conduct a biomechanical analysis to identify your unique pattern of muscle imbalances. By utilizing a series of muscle balance and motion analysis tests, we can identify the exact type, extent, and location of soft-tissue restrictions.

We then use ART treatments and follow-up exercises to release and resolve these restrictions, and then strengthen the muscles to prevent re-injury. With ART, we can look beyond just the symptomatic areas, and also consider the effect that other soft-tissue structures within the elbow's kinetic chain have upon the injury. These areas can include restrictions in structures ranging from the neck to the wrist.

ART achieves its high level of success because it can address and remove the multiple levels of restrictions that inhibit the translation and movement of soft-tissues.

A Case History - Elbow Injuries

Golfer's Elbow can be a very aggravating condition for the golf enthusiast (fanatic). A patient of mine, George, is just such a golfer. Newly retired, George played at least 10 rounds of 18-hole golf every week. George's wife refers to herself as a *golf widow,* one whose husband rises from the dead each spring.

Just one year after retirement, George developed a severe case of Golfer's Elbow (medial epicondylitis). When George came into our office, he was extremely upset; in fact, you would have thought his world had come to an end! Due to his injury, he had reduced his golfing to just one extremely painful game a week.

George sought treatment fairly soon after the initial injury. He was already icing the area, stretching, and had received several treatments of ultrasound, cross-fiber massage, and anti-inflammatory medications. These therapies did give him some short-term relief, but every time he got back on the course, he felt the return of his excruciating pain.

George's case is especially interesting because I found, when I examined him, that the physical restrictions at the elbow were quite minor. They were the type of restrictions that I could clear up with just a few ART treatments.

After the usual physical, orthopedic, and neurological tests, I had George demonstrate his golf swing. The first thing that jumped out at me was his inability to rotate his spine and his hips. Imbalances in hip rotation are commonly associated with repetitive strain injuries to the back, shoulder, and elbows. Golfers who lack full spinal rotation will often overuse their shoulders to try to compensate for this lack of rotation.

An examination of George's shoulder showed that it was actually much more restricted than his elbow. So, in George's case, what initially appeared to be a case of Golfer's Elbow, turned out to be a problem with restricted rotation of the hips and spine. This restriction had affected his shoulder, which in turn resulted in stresses to his elbow.

This is actually quite a common scenario where the problems in the chief area of complaint were actually a result of muscular and biomechanical compensations to problems in other structures. I worked with George for a total of six treatments – only two of these treatments were for his elbow – with the main focus upon the soft-tissue structures of the shoulder and low back.

Within a very short period of time, an elated George was back to his 10 rounds a week. Even better, he found that his game had improved substantially, much to the dismay of his wife. So much so that his wife has repeatedly asked if there was some way to get George to re-injure himself so that she could have more time with him!

Exercises for Resolving Elbow Injuries

Once the restrictions and adhesed tissues have been released with ART, post-treatment exercises become a critical part of the healing process, and act to ensure the elbow injury does not return.

It is important to remember that these exercises are only effective if they are executed *after* the adhesions within the soft-tissue have been released by ART treatments.

Attempts to stretch muscles that are currently bound by adhesions often do not achieve the desired results. In addition, only the muscles above and below the restrictions are lengthened. The actual restricted area remains unaffected, causing further muscle imbalances and stress, resulting in the formation of yet more restrictive tissues. This is why generic stretching exercises for elbow injuries seldom work.

In addition to stretching, a program of strengthening is also very important to ensure the problem does not return. The following pages depict some of the specific strengthening and stretching exercises that we recommend at our clinic for the prevention of elbow injuries.

- *Triceps Towel Stretch - page 69.*

- *Biceps and Pectoral Stretch - page 70.*

- *Biceps Curl - page 71.*

- *Loading the Triceps - page 72.*

Triceps Towel Stretch. This is an excellent stretching exercise that works a number of muscles including: triceps, subscapularis, serratus anterior, infraspinatus, teres minor, and teres major. You will need a long towel to do this exercise.

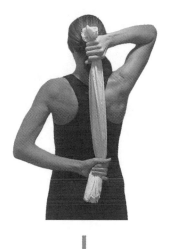

1. Stretch the towel, behind your back, holding both ends firmly.
   - The bottom hand should be at the small of the back.
   - The top hand should be behind the head.
2. Keep the bottom hand relaxed.
3. With the upper hand, slowly pull the towel upwards as far as you can comfortably stretch.
   - Take at least 30 seconds to reach this maximum stretch.
4. Now relax the *upper hand*.
5. With the lower hand, slowly pull the towel downwards as far as you can comfortably stretch.
   - Take at least 30 seconds to reach this maximum stretch.
6. Repeat this exercise five times, taking at least 30 seconds for each stretch.
7. Repeat the entire sequence for the other side.

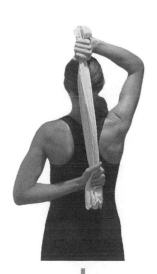

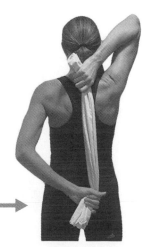

Biceps and Pectoral Stretch - This exercise lengthens the anterior aspects of the shoulder, as well as the biceps, and pectorals of the chest.

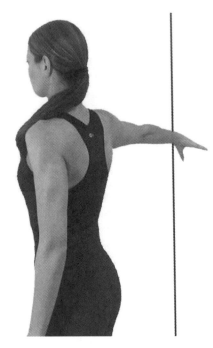

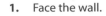

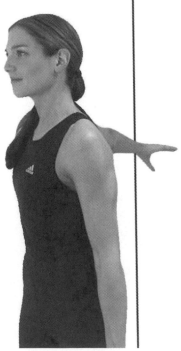

1. Face the wall.

2. Extend your arm, placing the edge of your hand against the wall, with your thumb pointing down to the floor.

3. With your hand on the wall, try to rotate the opposite shoulder and torso away from the wall.

4. Hold this stretch for 30 seconds or until the tension is released.

   You should feel a light tension in the shoulder, biceps, and chest.

5. Repeat this stretch once for each side.

Biceps Curl. This exercise strengthens your biceps. It focuses upon correct activation and strengthening of the muscles. Use a weight which causes you to *lose* good form after 10 to 12 repetitions. This indicates that you are actually working the muscle to its full capacity.

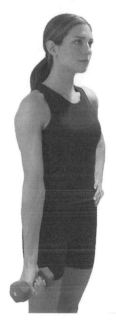
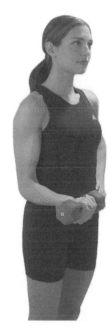
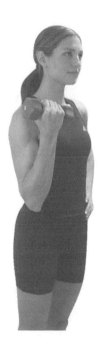

1. Stand straight with your arms by your side in neutral position, with the weight in your affected hand. Keep your chin and chest high.

2. Curl the arm upwards until your forearm is parallel to the floor.

3. Curl up for a count of 1, and slowly down for a count of 3.
   You want a quick contraction, and a slow return to starting position. Your palm should always be facing upwards.

4. Repeat this exercise 10 to 12 times, for three sets.

5. Repeat this exercise for exactly the same number of times for the strong side.

Loading the Triceps. This exercise focuses upon strengthening the extensors of the elbow through all its ranges of motion. Use a weight which causes your triceps to tire after 10 to 12 repetitions. This indicates that you are actually working the muscle to its full capacity. Ideally, you should start with a light weight of 5 to 8 pounds, and build up from there.

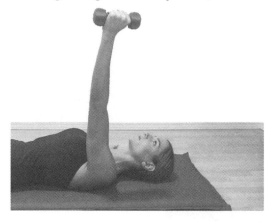

1. Lie down on your back with your knees bent.

2. Hold the weight in your affected hand and raise your arm so that it is perpendicular to the ceiling, and your palm is facing to the side.

3. Bend your elbow to lower the weight down in an arc that ends by touching your shoulder. Lower for a slow count of 4.

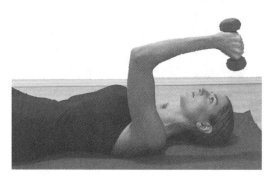

4. Bring the weight back up to its original position - within a count of 2. You want a slow contraction, and a quicker return to starting position.

5. Repeat this exercise 12 to 15 times, for 1 to 3 sets. Your triceps should fatigue within this repetition range if you are using the correct weight.

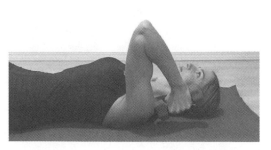

6. Repeat for the *same* number of repetitions with the strong side.

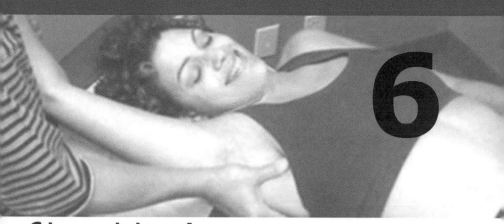

Shoulder Injuries

In this chapter

Ask yourself:

■ Do you have shoulder pain that increased gradually over time?

■ Have you ever had an injury to your shoulder?

■ Do you have pain when you raise or rotate your arms? Can you rotate your arm and shoulder through all its normal positions?

■ Does it feel like your shoulder could pop out or slide out of the socket?

■ Do you lack the strength in your shoulder to carry out your daily activities?

■ Do you have pain at night that prevents you from sleeping on the affected side?

If you answered YES to one or more of the above questions, you may be suffering from a soft-tissue injury to the muscles and tissues of your shoulder. Common shoulder syndromes include Tendonitis, Bursitis, Rotator Cuff Injury and Frozen Shoulder – which can often be effectively treated with Active Release Techniques (ART).

What Causes Shoulder Injuries?

Our shoulders are designed to provide an optimum range of motion – at the cost of stability. Compared to other joints in our bodies the shoulder joint is quite *unstable*. When shoulder injuries occur, this inherent instability immediately affects a variety of anatomical structures within the shoulder's kinetic chain.

Shoulder injuries, like many repetitive stress injuries, usually develop over long periods of time. The muscles and soft-tissues of the shoulder can be stressed by:

■ Increased physical activity.

■ Acute and repeated trauma to the shoulder.

■ Repetitive actions that involve shoulder movement.

■ Existing muscle imbalances.

■ Soft-tissue restrictions in structures ranging from the shoulder through to the structures in the shoulder's kinetic chain (arm, back, and neck).

■ Scar tissue generated as a result of surgical procedures.

Like all other repetitive strain injuries, these varied stresses cause the body to lay down restrictive adhesive fibers between muscle layers in an attempt to protect the stressed tissues. Unfortunately, these adhesions also bind together the layers of muscles and soft-tissues, and prevent them from moving freely, thereby restricting their function.

These restrictions, in turn, affect the function and strength of other structures within the shoulder's kinetic chain. By considering kinetic chain relationships, we can see how a single shoulder dysfunction can soon lead to a series of other physical dysfunctions in the back, neck, and arms.

Who suffers from shoulder injuries?

Shoulder injuries can be caused by repetitive actions that occur in a broad range of activities and sports. Shoulder injuries often occur in:

• Assembly Line Workers
• Baseball Players
• Basketball Players
• Computer Operators
• Construction Workers
• Cashiers
• Dental Assistants
• Dentists
• Football Players
• Golfers
• Hairdressers
• Painters
• Postal Workers
• Racquet Sports Players
• Rugby Players
• Skiers
• Sports involving throwing
• Swimmers
• Tennis Players
• Weightlifters

74

About the Shoulder

The shoulder joint (glenohumeral joint) is a ball and socket joint which joins the upper body to the arm. The shoulder joint is made up of three osseous structures, and several soft-tissue structures:

■ Clavicle, or collarbone.

■ Scapula, or shoulder blade.

■ Humerus, a bone located in your upper arm which articulates with the scapula at the shoulder and with bones of the forearm at the elbow.

■ Rotator cuff muscles and ligaments.

■ Tendons which attach the muscles to the bones.

■ Ligaments which attach bones to bones, and help to keep the shoulder in place.

■ Bursa, a fluid-filled sac between the shoulder joint and the rotator cuff, which acts to prevent the rotator cuff from rubbing against the shoulder.

The muscles, soft-tissues, and bones of the shoulder create a balance of forces that provide both mobility and stability. When this balance is disrupted, the shoulder becomes prone to injury and dysfunction.

It is essential to understand the inter-relationships, relative motions, and links between these various soft-tissue structures before trying to resolve any shoulder problems. See the following topics for more details about the structure of the shoulder:

■ *Rotator Cuff Muscles - page 76.*

■ *Scapula or Shoulder Blade - page 77.*

■ *Other Muscles of the Shoulder - page 78.*

Note: Many patients manifest the *same physical pain symptoms*, but have different soft-tissue structures causing the problem. The location and type of pain symptoms do *not* indicate which soft-tissue structure is damaged, or which is the cause of the problem.

The only way to determine exactly which soft-tissue structures are involved is by '*feeling*' where the restrictions are located. Qualified ART practitioners, with their highly-developed sense of touch, are able to find and identify the specific soft-tissues that are affected, and then remove the restrictive adhesions from these soft-tissues to restore full function.

Rotator Cuff Muscles

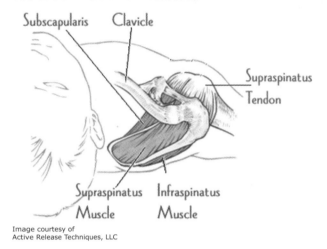

Subscapularis   Clavicle

Supraspinatus
Tendon

Supraspinatus   Infraspinatus
Muscle   Muscle

Image courtesy of
Active Release Techniques, LLC

The rotator cuff is made up of four major muscles and their associated tendons: supraspinatus, infraspinatus, teres minor, and the subscapularis. The rotator cuff muscles:

- Are used to generate torque for shoulder movement.
- Act as dynamic stabilizers of the shoulder joint (glenohumeral joint).
- Help to lower and stabilize the humeral head (end of the humerus bone) that fits into the shoulder joint.

A restriction, shortening, or change in length of any one of these muscles can immediately affect the balance, movement, and function of the shoulder.

Rotator cuff injuries are the common consequence of repetitive overhead activities such as tennis, swimming, baseball, and weight-training. Chronic pain in any sport that involves reaching overhead is often the result of damage to the rotator-cuff muscles.

See *Rotator Cuff, Impingements & Tendonitis - page 80* for more information about how restrictions and impingements in this area can affect shoulder function, and to understand how these problems can be resolved.

Scapula or Shoulder Blade

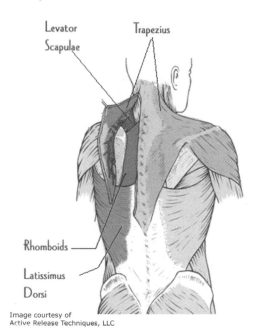

Levator Scapulae

Trapezius

Rhomboids

Latissimus Dorsi

Image courtesy of
Active Release Techniques, LLC

The scapula acts as a fulcrum for muscles that control shoulder motion. Almost all shoulder and arm motions are greatly influenced by the mobility of the scapula.

For example: As you raise your arm from your side, the scapula rotates one degree for every two degrees of motion of the arm. This means that any soft-tissue restrictions that inhibit the motion of the scapula will *directly* affect your ability to raise and lower your arm.

The scapula is often considered to be the foundation or base for the soft-tissue structures of the upper body. Fifteen major muscles attach to the scapula, of which nine help to control shoulder motion. The other six muscles are involved with supporting the scapula itself. Shoulder dysfunctions can occur whenever there is any restriction or injury to the muscles attached to the scapula.

Restrictions in soft-tissues attached to the scapula immediately affect the performance of all other soft-tissue structures within the scapula's kinetic chain. These key muscles include the:

- Trapezius.
- Levator Scapulae.
- Rhomboids.
- Teres Minor and Teres Major.
- Latissimus Dorsi.
- All antagonistic or opposing muscles.

To properly restore function and relieve pain, all of these associated structures and the muscles of the scapula must also be evaluated and treated.

Other Muscles of the Shoulder

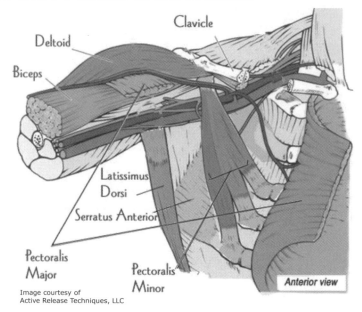

Clavicle

Deltoid

Biceps

Latissimus Dorsi

Serratus Anterior

Pectoralis Major

Pectoralis Minor

Anterior view

Image courtesy of
Active Release Techniques, LLC

Muscles such as the serratus anterior, pectoralis minor, pectoralis major, and latissimus dorsi all play a *counterbalancing* role in the performance of shoulder movements and are critical for optimal control and balance of the shoulder. For example, the anterior pectoralis muscles help to counterbalance the actions of the posterior muscles of the rhomboids and trapezius.

Restrictions in any of the soft-tissues of the shoulder will always affect the function of the counterbalancing tissues on the other side.   New adhesions may be laid down to compensate for these additional stresses.

Biomechanical imbalances often occur with weightlifting. Many weight programs put too much emphasis on pushing movements. This problem is commonly seen with routines that put an emphasis on the bench press, an exercise which stresses the pectoralis muscles. However, most of these programs do *not* balance the effects of this action with exercises that strengthen the rhomboids and trapezius, the muscles that act as the counterbalance for the pectoralis muscles.

Practitioners must consider and remove restrictions in both the primary movers and their counterbalancing muscles in order to effectively resolve shoulder problems.

The Traditional Perspective

Typical traditional methods generally require a long period of time before they can provide significant relief from the pain caused by the physical restrictions. Unfortunately, this relief is generally temporary in nature, and symptoms typically return within a short time.

Traditional treatment methods for frozen shoulder, tendonitis, bursitis, and rotator cuff injuries deliver relatively poor *symptomatic* relief, require a long period of treatment, and provide only temporary solutions to the problem. Most of these techniques use indirect methods in an attempt to restore mobility to the shoulder joint, but do not address or resolve the true cause of the problem - the restrictive adhesions between tissue layers. These traditional treatment methods generally *fail* to resolve the shoulder injury because they:

- Only treat the *symptoms* rather than the *cause* of injury. For example, medication provides symptomatic relief by hiding the pain caused by a compressed or impinged nerve, but it does not release the impingement. The medication provides *symptomatic relief* by hiding the pain signals.

- Do not remove or resolve the root cause of the shoulder injury – the restrictive connective fibers that bind and restrict the inflamed soft-tissues.

- Do not resolve the problems and restrictions in adjacent structures that may actually be the root cause of the problem. These other structures in the shoulder's kinetic chain may also be restricted or damaged, and must also be treated for full problem resolution.

Traditional Treatments

Many of the following traditional methods are important aspects of the overall treatment strategy - but often only provide temporary *symptomatic* relief.

- Anti-inflammatory drugs
- Ice
- Rest
- Stretching
- Electric modalities
- Exercises
- Surgery
- Steroid Injections
- Ultrasound

Problems with Tradition

- Repeated use of steroids weakens tendons, resulting in further biomechanical imbalances in the shoulder.
- Most traditional treatments provide only *symptomatic* relief from the pain.
- Most traditional treatments do not remove the restrictive adhesions that are the true cause of the problem.

About Symptomatic Relief

Symptomatic Relief describes treatments that take away or hide the signs or signals of the problem.

These treatments alleviate the patient's perception of pain, without dealing with the underlying cause of the problem.

Rotator Cuff, Impingements & Tendonitis

Injuries to the rotator cuff and its tendons are very common in the workplace and in the athletic arena, and can affect all age groups.

Repetitive stresses to the shoulder can cause the following types of injuries:

- A tear or injury to the muscles and tendons of the rotator cuff.

- Impingement or pinching of the rotator cuff between the shoulder joint and the overlying bony protuberance – the acromion.

- Bursitis – inflammation of the bursa – usually caused by frequent extension of the arm at high speeds, such as in painting, hanging wallpaper, or drapes, washing windows.

- Tendonitis or inflammation of the rotator cuff tendons caused by aggressive overuse of weak muscles.

These syndromes are typically characterized by the following symptoms:

- Shoulder pain when moving the shoulder, or when sleeping on it.

- Tenderness and weakness in the shoulder.

- Lack of mobility in the shoulder.

- Recurrent, constant pain, particularly with activities where the arm is overhead for long periods of time.

- Muscle weakness, especially when attempting to lift the arm.

- Catching, grating or cracking sounds when the arm is moved.

- Limited motion of the shoulder and arm.

What causes these shoulder injuries?

Rotator Cuff, Impingement, and Tendonitis injuries of the shoulder are caused by a variety of activities including:

- Repetitive actions that stress the shoulder.

- Intense overhead motions.

- Heavy lifting activities.

- Repetitive overhead motions such as pitching a ball or painting a ceiling.

- Excessive force or trauma caused by a fall or accident.

- Degeneration due to aging or poor posture and weak muscles.

- A reduction in blood supply to the shoulder tendons.

- Narrowing of the space (acromioclavicular arch) between the collarbone (clavicle) and the top portion (acromion) of the shoulder blade (scapula).

- Abrasion, impingement, or rubbing of the surface of the rotator cuff by the top portion of the shoulder blade.

These repetitive stresses cause microtrauma to the soft-tissues of the shoulder, lead to tissue inflammation, cause formation of restrictive adhesions that bind and restrict tissue layers, and result in shortened and weakened muscles. Traditional treatments rarely completely resolve these conditions.

Active Release Techniques takes a very different approach for treating rotator cuff, impingement, and tendonitis injuries. ART considers the unique restrictions that can occur in each shoulder injury, as well as the impact of those injuries upon other soft-tissue structures along the shoulder's entire kinetic chain.

This complete evaluation is very important since any restriction, adhesion, or lack of translation in the rotator cuff greatly affects its function, and that of its associated soft-tissue structures.

For example, consider how a restriction of the subscapularis (one of the muscles in the rotator cuff) affects shoulder function:

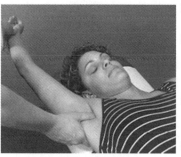

Dr. Abelson removing restrictions from the subscapularis muscle.

- The subscapularis is located on the anterior (front) side of the scapula.
- The subscapularis muscle acts to *internally* rotate your shoulder and pulls the shoulder and arm *toward* the body.
- When restrictions occur in the subscapularis, you are unable to lift your shoulder and/or arm.
- Restrictions in the subscapularis affect the biomechanics of the scapula's counterbalancing muscles. These can also restrict motion, resulting in decreased shoulder motion.

Each and every structure in the rotator cuff muscle needs to be evaluated for relative translation, and if restricted, that muscle must be released in order to return full function to the shoulder.

Frozen Shoulder

Frozen Shoulder, or adhesive capsulitis, is a general term used to describe all injuries that result in a *loss of motion* to the shoulder. This is a very debilitating and restrictive condition which affects all activities of daily living. Frozen Shoulder is characterized by:

■ Loss of motion in the shoulder joint.

■ Difficulties in raising the arm above the head, across the body, or behind the back.

The actual cause of this condition is unknown, but Frozen Shoulder commonly occurs after:

■ Prolonged immobilization.

■ A history of trauma or a previous surgery to the shoulder.

■ An inflammation of shoulder tissues where the capsule surrounding the shoulder joint thickens and contracts. This inflammation leaves less space for the upper arm bone (humerus) to move around.

Traditional treatments include:

■ Standard pain medications.

■ Muscle relaxants.

■ Heat and ice therapies.

■ Corticosteroid injections.

■ Exercises.

Most of these therapies are ineffective and slow to achieve results, with any type of resolution taking anywhere from *twelve to forty-two weeks*. They fail because they do not work directly on the affected tissues, but only concentrate upon providing symptomatic relief. In addition, the majority of traditional therapies only concentrate on increasing the range-of-motion through indirect procedures and exercises, rather than working directly on the affected soft-tissue structures.

Active Release Techniques, on the other hand, is very effective in treating and resolving this condition. Most cases treated at our office show an 80% improvement within three weeks. This condition can take longer to respond to treatments than other soft-tissue injuries, but the duration of treatment with ART is still very short compared to other therapies.

ART is able to achieve this remarkable success rate due to its direct approach in treating the shoulder's joint capsule and its associated soft-tissues. ART literally strips away the restrictions that bind soft-tissue layers together to restore mobility and translation to affected tissues.

Using ART's direct approach for the treatment of Frozen Shoulder, we look for restrictions in all the soft-tissues of the shoulder, as well as in the shoulder's kinetic chain, and then treat all required areas. These muscles can include:

- Subscapularis.
- Supraspinatus.
- Subclavius.
- Infraspinatus.

See *page 76* for a detailed image of these structures. In addition, muscles in the back or posterior of the shoulder must be addressed, including:

- Deltoid muscles.
- Teres major.
- Teres minor.

Posterior View of the Shoulder

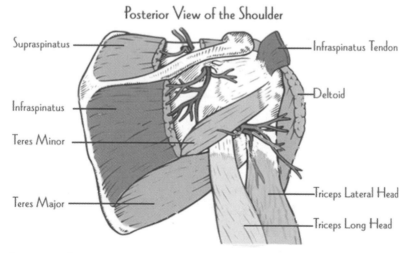

Image courtesy of Active Release Techniques, LLC

And finally, the opposing muscles at the front of the shoulder including all aspects of the glenohumeral joint capsule, pectoralis major, and pectoralis minor must be addressed. See *page 78* for a detailed image.

ART - A Better Solution

Effective treatment of shoulder problems, or of any soft-tissue injury (ligaments, muscles, blood vessels, fascia and nerves), requires an alteration in tissue structure to:

- Break up the restrictive cross-fiber adhesions.
- Restore normal tissue translation and movement.
- Restore strength, flexibility, balance, and stability to the affected soft-tissues.

As we have seen, the shoulder is composed of numerous layers of muscles, tendons, nerves, and other soft-tissues. When the shoulder becomes injured, the practitioner needs an effective means to identify exactly *which* structures are actually injured.

For example, when a patient tells us that a part of her shoulder really hurts, we need to be able to determine if the injury was at the tissues on the surface (superficial) or if the injury lies deeper within the tissue layers, or perhaps even further down the shoulder's kinetic chain in a structure which is not currently in pain.

The ART practitioner's highly-developed sense of touch lets him or her locate the affected tissue layer by *feeling* the adhesions, *finding* the restricted tissues, and then physically *working* the restricted area back to its normal texture, tension, and length by using various soft-tissue manipulation methods.
Active Release Techniques is very successful at treating shoulder injuries because it:

- Substantially decreases healing time for most shoulder injuries, with noticeable positive results within a few weeks of treatment.
- Treats the root cause of the injury by removing the restrictive adhesions between both the superficial and deep tissue areas. These adhesions restrict soft-tissue translation and movement, and prevent full range of motion of the shoulder. Most other shoulder treatments only address the area that is manifesting pain, and do not always address the tissues that are truly causing the problem.
- Treats restricted or bound tissues along the entire kinetic chain of the shoulder. This kinetic chain can involve many areas that are not part of the shoulder. For example, shoulder injuries in

golfers are often due to the compensation the body must make when there is a lack of spinal rotation. Unless the restrictions in spinal rotation are removed, the shoulder problems will never be completely resolved.

■ Improves strength, flexibility, endurance, and overall athletic performance.

Athletes ranging from weekend warriors to Olympic gold medalists have seen substantial performance improvements after receiving ART treatments.

■ Even improves your golf game after the first few visits. My patients often joke that it would have been cheaper and more effective for them to have seen me first, instead of buying that expensive high-tech driver.

A Case History

Frozen Shoulder can be an extremely exasperating and painful condition for the patient. Many of our patients come to us in a last-ditch effort to avoid surgery.

A classic case of frozen shoulder occurred with Jean. Jean works as an executive for an oil and gas company. Jean showed all the classical signs and symptoms of frozen shoulder:

■ A slow onset of the condition.

■ Pain near the insertion of the deltoid muscle.

■ An inability to sleep on her affected side.

A Patient's Story...

I had been experiencing pain in my neck and right shoulder since 1990 (at age 34).

The problem was not caused by a specific single injury, but by extensive computer work. I had been working on a computer since 1987 (full time) and the work escalated in 1990 when I became a legal assistant for a major real estate developer in Montreal. At the time, the recommended treatment by my family doctor was physiotherapy and NSAID (non-steroidal anti-inflammatory drugs) therapy. Neither were very helpful in relieving the pain.

Shortly thereafter, I tried regular chiropractic treatments (only spinal adjustments) and this did not help either.

Over the course of the many following years, I tried the following treatments:

• Sports therapy at a University in Montreal (which in retrospect was very similar to ART) and this seemed to help a little.

• Physiotherapy.

• Massage Therapy.

• Chiropractic Therapy.

• Prolotherapy, a very painful procedure which did not help at all - if anything made it worse.

- Pain and restriction on elevation and external rotation of her arm.
- Completely normal X-rays.

Unfortunately for Jean, both sides of her shoulders were affected by this problem. Frozen Shoulder wasn't Jean's only concern. Jean has been a diabetic since the age of seven. (About 42% of patients who suffer bilateral frozen shoulder are diabetic.[1])

Before coming to our clinic, Jean had already tried numerous therapies, all with little positive effect. These included:

- Physiotherapy for 2 months, at 3 times per week.
- Steroid injections.
- Chiropractic.
- Acupuncture.
- Massage.
- Exercise programs.

When nothing else works, conventional treatment sometimes recommends manipulation under anaesthesia. (In very rare cases, where the patient does not respond to ART treatments, we may recommend this procedure.) In Jean's case, her medical doctor advised against this due to the poor response many diabetics have when this procedure is used.

Our physical examination revealed some interesting points. Jean showed:

- Severe restrictions in her shoulders.
- Very poor circulation from her shoulders right down to her hands.

A Patient's Story...(continued)

Finally, I heard of ART and then someone recommended Dr. Abelson to me.

I began ART treatments in 1999 and they helped almost immediately. I had regular treatments for a few weeks and then was able to go for periodic treatments at one-month intervals.

My enjoyment of life has improved about 80% since ART. I am able to continue to work 50 hours / week at a very demanding job (which I enjoy) and this too I believe is thanks to ART.

I have recommended the treatment to friends and family and will continue to do so because of the pain relief that I have experienced.

Dr. Abelson seems to be able to find the "tight" spots and provides immediate relief to the affected area. The bonus is that ART is the least invasive treatment for pain - AND IT WORKS!

**Linda Nussbaum,
Executive Assistant
The Forzani Group Ltd.**

---

1. Orthoteers- Frozen Shoulder, http://www.orthoteers.co.uk/ Nrujp~ij33lm/Orthshouldfrozen.htm

- Severe soft-tissue restriction in her hands, wrists, forearms, elbows, and neck.

- Restrictions in her hands that were so severe that she was starting to have trouble closing her hands.

Palpation of her arm and hand showed that Jean had literally lost most normal tissue translation from her hands right up to her neck.

ART uses a very direct approach for treating Frozen Shoulder. While ART treatments always address *all* the soft-tissue structures (muscles, ligaments, tendons, fascia) that may be involved, our primary work focused directly on the rotator cuff joint capsule.

Jean found the first few ART treatments to be quite painful. The restrictions were so hard, and the tissues so tight, that it was difficult for me to access the structures that needed to be treated. However, Jean was willing to put up with the short-term pain if we could provide good long-term results.

In Jean's case, it took about eight visits before seeing a 90% improvement in her condition. These are remarkable results when one considers the severity of her restrictions, and the length of time in which these restrictions had been building up.

We were also able to resolve her neck, arm, wrist, and hand pain in this short time period. In fact, after the first treatment, Jean was able to close her hands completely – something she had been unable to do for several years.

Other procedures use an indirect approach – hoping to stretch the joint capsule by using shoulder joint motions. This indirect approach is often very slow at achieving any results.

Previous to using the ART approach, it would have taken me months to achieve any type of positive results for a case such as this one. Now, with ART, we are able to provide a more permanent resolution to the problem within a relatively short time.

Exercises for the Shoulder

The inherent instability of the shoulder requires us to maintain a strong, balanced shoulder to both prevent injuries and to allow for optimum performance with any sport or other daily activities.

Once the restrictions and adhesed tissues have been released with ART, post-treatment exercises become a critical part of the healing process, and act to ensure the shoulder injury does not return.

It is important to remember that exercises are only effective if they are executed *after* the adhesions within the soft-tissue have been released by ART treatments.

Attempts to stretch muscles that are currently bound by adhesions often do not achieve the desired results. In addition, only the muscles above and below the restrictions are lengthened. The actual restricted area remains unaffected, causing further muscle imbalances and stresses, and resulting in the formation of yet more restrictive tissues. This is why generic stretching exercises for shoulder injuries seldom work.

In addition to stretching, a program of strengthening is also very important to ensure the problem does not return. The following pages depict some of the specific strengthening and stretching exercises that we recommend at our clinic for the prevention of shoulder injuries.

- *Setting and Activating the Scapula - page 89.*
- *Building Awareness of the Lower Trapezius Muscles - page 90.*
- *Triceps Towel Stretch - page 91.*
- *Ball Hold Against the Wall - page 92.*
- *Strengthening the External Rotators of the Shoulder - page 93.*
- *Strengthening the Serratus Anterior and Lower Trapezius - page 94.*

Setting and Activating the Scapula - This exercise helps you to build awareness of where the scapula is and learn what its normal positioning should be. You will need this awareness to do the remainder of the exercises in this chapter. Always start with this exercise.

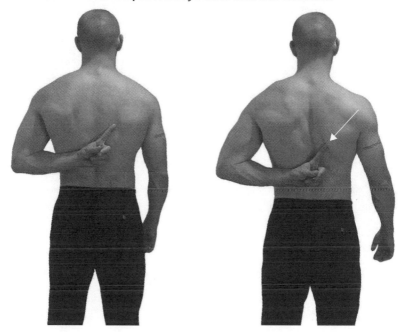

1. Stand straight, with both hands hanging loosely by your sides.

2. Take your right hand, and with your forefinger, reach behind your back to lightly touch the medial (bottom inner) edge of your left scapula.

3. Keep the other arm relaxed.

4. Bring your scapula downwards and towards the midline of your back to activate the lower trapezius muscles. You should be pushing towards the finger that is touching the scapula.

    Ensure you do not activate any other muscles. Keep the upper trapezius and latissimus dorsi of the back quiet. The entire movement should come from the muscles (lower trapezius) pushing the scapula down onto the finger.

    This is the scapula's *normal* (and desired) position for many of the exercises in this chapter.

5. Hold this position for 3 to 5 seconds and then take 3 to 5 seconds to release and return to neutral position.

6. Repeat this movement 10 times for each side.

Building Awareness of the Lower Trapezius Muscles - The lower trapezius muscle contributes both strength and stability to the shoulders. It needs to be in structural balance to reduce chances of injury, and to ensure proper recovery from shoulder injuries. You must first complete the *Setting and Activating the Scapula - page 89* exercise before beginning this exercise.

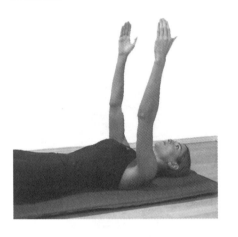

1. Lie flat on your back and reset your scapulae to the normal position. (See "Setting and Activating the Scapula" - page 89, for details.)

2. Raise your arms so that they are perpendicular to the ground.

3. Close your eyes, and **very slowly** lower your arms, over your head towards the ground.

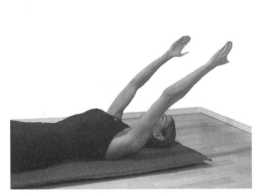

4. Take at least 30 seconds to slowly lower your arms to the ground.

5. Ensure your scapula stays on the floor for the entire motion.
   Stop the motion when your scapulae start to lift off the ground or when you start to use your upper trapezius muscle.

6. Check your range of motion.

7. Repeat this exercise 5 times, taking at least 30 seconds for each repetition. Your range of motion should increase slightly with each repetition.

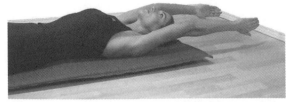

Triceps Towel Stretch - This is an excellent stretching exercise that works a number of muscles including: triceps, subscapularis, serratus anterior, infraspinatus, teres minor, and teres major. You will need a long towel to do this exercise.

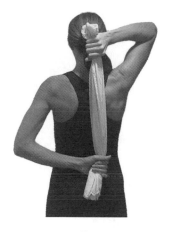

1. Stretch the towel behind your back, holding both ends firmly.
   - The bottom hand should be at the small of the back.
   - The top hand should be behind the head.
2. Keep the bottom hand relaxed.
3. With the upper hand, slowly pull the towel upwards as far as you can comfortably stretch.
   - Take at least 30 seconds to reach this maximum stretch.
4. Now relax the *upper hand*.
5. With the lower hand, slowly pull the towel downwards as far as you can comfortably stretch.
   - Take at least 30 seconds to reach this maximum stretch.
6. Repeat this exercise five times, taking at least 30 seconds for each stretch.
7. Repeat the entire sequence for the other side.

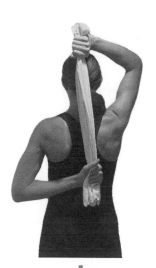

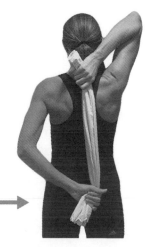

Ball Hold Against the Wall - This exercise works on your proprioception, balance, and coordination for the shoulder and its surrounding muscles. Most people will require a 55cm exercise ball.

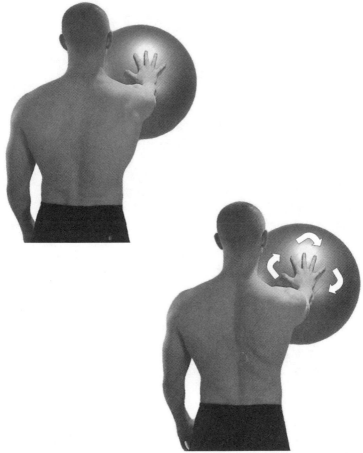

1.   Place the ball against the wall – at about face height – and hold it there with one hand.

2.   Set your scapula to its *normal* position, using the method described in *Setting and Activating the Scapula - page 89.*

3.   Roll 10-15 small circles with the ball against the wall – while keeping the scapula set.

   ■   Make sure you do *not* activate or use the upper trapezius.
   ■   Avoid shrugging.

4.   Repeat this exercise, rolling 10-15 circles, in the *opposite* direction.

Strengthening the External Rotators of the Shoulder - You will need a 5-to-8 lb. hand weight for this exercise. This exercise develops shoulder strength and coordination, and is important for developing upper body structural balance in the shoulder joint.

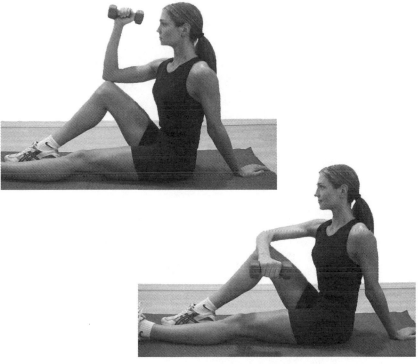

1. Sit on the floor, with the strong hand resting on the ground, and the opposite knee bent.

2. Pick up the weight with your affected arm and prop this arm on the raised knee. Your arm should be bent at the elbow at 90 degrees, pointing up to the ceiling.

3. Keep your arm at 90 degrees and lower it to a count of 3 slowly towards the ground until the forearm is parallel to the ground.

4. Rotate back to the starting position - without pausing. Raise to a count of 2.

5. Repeat this exercise 12 to 20 times - depending on your strength. If the weight is correct, you should be able to execute at least 12 repetitions of these exercises, and feel fatigue within 12 to 20 repetitions.

6. Repeat this exercise for your strong side – for exactly the same number of repetitions. Do not exceed this number since you are attempting to balance the two sides of your body.

7. Perform 1 to 3 sets each time.

Strengthening the Serratus Anterior and Lower Trapezius -

This exercise is useful for building strength and coordination in the muscles that work together in the shoulder joint. This exercise requires the use of an elastic band or tubing.

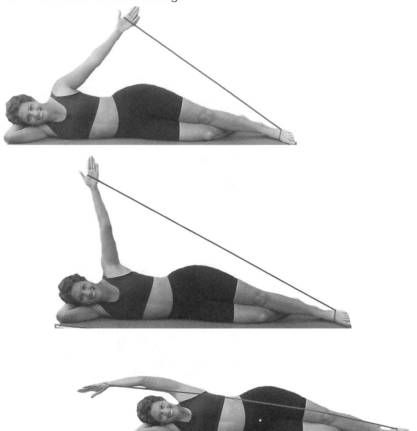

1. Lie on the ground on your strong side.

2. Attach the tubing to the hand on the affected side and to your upper foot.

3. Pull your arm over your head to stretch the band as far as you can while keeping the lower trapezius muscles activated.

4. Raise and stretch the hand for a count of 5 seconds, and then lower your hand for another count of 5 seconds.

5. Repeat this exercise 6 to 10 times for your weak side.

6. Repeat this exercise for your strong side – for exactly the same number of repetitions. Do not exceed this number since you are attempting to balance the two sides of your body. Perform 1 to 3 sets each time.

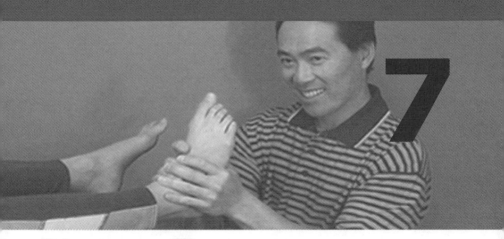

Plantar Fasciitis

In this chapter

Ask yourself:

- Do you experience heel pain with the first few steps of the morning?
- Do you have pain at the center of the heel when you place weight on your foot?
- Do you experience dull aching or sharp, burning pain in your heel?
- Do you feel a pulling sensation in your heel?

If you answered YES to one or more of the above questions, you may have *Plantar Fasciitis* - also commonly diagnosed as *Heel Spurs*. Unfortunately, this diagnosis is nonspecific and inaccurate and commonly leads to the application of a wide range of ineffective treatments.

Plantar Fasciitis, in the majority of cases, can be effectively treated with Active Release Techniques.

What is Plantar Fasciitis?

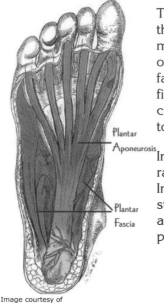

Plantar Aponeurosis

Plantar Fascia

Image courtesy of
Active Release Techniques, LLC

The term "itis" means inflammation. In the medical literature, Plantar Fasciitis is most often described as an inflammation of the plantar aponeuroisis or plantar fascia. The plantar fascia is a thin band of fibrous tissue that runs from the calcaneus (heel bone) to the base of the toes.

Interestingly, the actual plantar fascia is rarely tender to palpation and touch. Instead, it is the deeper soft-tissue structures that show signs of tenderness, and that cause the actual pain felt by patients.

What Causes Plantar Fasciitis?

Plantar Fasciitis, like all repetitive stress injuries, typically develops over a long period of time. The fascia and soft-tissues of the feet can be stressed by:

- Alterations in normal foot biomechanics due to physical activity.
- Soft-tissue restrictions in tissues ranging from the foot to the hamstrings.
- Repetitive motions that stress soft-tissues in the feet and legs.
- Standing on hard surfaces for long periods of time.
- Existing muscle imbalances.
- Increased physical activity.
- Shoes that do not provide arch support.
- Acute trauma to the feet.

As a result of these repeated stresses, the fascia and surrounding tissues develop micro-tears. When these tissues lack the time or opportunity to heal properly, they become inflamed and irritated by their continual usage.

The inflammation process causes the body to lay down additional restrictive, adhesive scar tissue across the inflamed structures, and results in a shortening of the *plantar aponeurosis*.

These restrictive fibers also bind the layers of adjacent soft-tissues together, and prevent them from translating or moving freely across each other. This entrapment causes further friction and inflammation. Ultrasound measurements from tissues of symptomatic and non-symptomatic patients showed the symptomatic tissue to have an increased thickening, as the various soft-tissue layers adhered together.[1]

Are Heel Spurs the Cause of Plantar Fasciitis?

Standard medical literature often uses the term '*heel spurs*' synonymously to describe plantar fasciitis. This usage is both confusing and misleading since heel spurs:

- Are actually spike-like projections of new bone that do not usually cause pain.
- Are only formed *after* the plantar aponeurosis becomes inflamed.
- Have been shown to be a side-effect or result of the actual problem – inflammation of several layers of deep tissue in the foot that have become adhesed together.
- Continue to exist, and can be seen in X-rays, even after the Plantar Fasciitis problem is fully resolved.
- Cause no pain and are incidental to the cause or resolution of Plantar Fasciitis.

Who suffers from Plantar Fasciitis?

Plantar Fasciitis is caused by repetitive actions such as those experienced by:

- Runners
- Walkers
- Football Players
- Cashiers
- Hairdressers
- Postal Workers
- Factory Workers
- Nurses

In addition, Plantar Fasciitis can be caused by:

- Flat or excessively high arches.
- Any situation that requires standing on hard surfaces.
- Sudden increases in physical activity.
- Being overweight.
- Weak foot muscles.
- Poor shoe support.
- Excessive foot pronation.

1. Wall, J., Harkness, M., & Cook, B. (1993). Ultrasound diagnosis of plantar fasciitis. Foot Ankle Int, 14(8), 465-470

The Traditional Perspective

The medical community has been arguing about the cause and solution for Plantar Fasciitis for over 200 years.[1]

Traditional treatment methods used over the last 200 years have continued to deliver relatively poor *symptomatic* relief. Unfortunately, many of these treatments leave patients unable to perform their daily activities without continuing to experience some degree of pain.

Typical traditional treatments can take 6 to 12 months before they provide any level of relief from the pain. Unfortunately, this relief is generally temporary in nature, and symptoms typically return within a short time.

These traditional treatment methods fail to resolve Plantar Fasciitis since they:

- Treat only the *symptoms* rather than the *cause* of Plantar Fasciitis.
- Do not consider the deeper soft-tissue structures that may also be restricted or inflamed.
- Do not consider the other restrictions that may exist within the foot's kinetic chain – from the foot to the hamstrings.
- Do not remove or resolve the root cause of plantar fasciitis – the restrictive connective fibers that bind and restrict the inflamed soft-tissues.

Traditional Treatments for Plantar Fasciitis

Traditional treatments include:

- Ice
- Rest
- Stretching
- Massage
- Orthotics
- Ultrasound
- Anti-inflammatories
- Tapping
- Osseous adjustments

These procedures are all important aspects in the overall treatment strategy. But used on their own, each of these techniques only provides only temporary symptomatic relief.

Most of these techniques do *not* remove the true cause of the injury – the restrictive adhesions.

---

1. Chandler T, & Kibler W. (1993). A biomechanical approach to prevention, treatment and rehabilitation of plantar fasciitis. Sports Medicine, 15(5), 344-352.

ART - A Better Solution

Even though people will continue to argue about which is the most effective treatment for Plantar Fasciitis, we believe that the results that are achieved with ART speak for themselves. The best treatment results will be achieved by the therapy that addressees the true, root cause of the problem.

Standard treatment techniques generally achieve poor results since practitioners often do not consider the deeper soft-tissue structures which are also Involved in causing Plantar Fasciitis.

ART views Plantar Fasciitis as a series of soft-tissue restrictions that inhibit biomechanical motions. These restrictions limit tissue translation and affect the biomechanics of the entire body.

Our clinical experience has shown that Plantar Fasciitis is caused by *more* than just inflammation of the plantar aponeurosis. We have found that in addition to the inflammation of the plantar aponeurosis, we must also take into account:

- Two commonly-ignored deep muscles that lie below the plantar aponeurosis – the *quadratus plantae* and the *flexor digitorum brevis*.[1]
- The altered biomechanics caused by soft-tissue restrictions in other parts of the feet and legs.
- Layers of tissue deep within the foot that have lost their ability to translate or move freely across one another due to restrictive adhesions that formed between adjacent structures.

A Patient's Story....

Dear Dr. Abelson:

I wanted to let you know about my experience with Active Release Techniques (ART).

For many years I had suffered from Plantar Fasciitis on both of my feet. The pain would sometimes become unbearable. Although I wear orthotics, I could never quite get the relief I was looking for.

That is, until I heard about ART. After only three treatments with you, I received significant relief from the pain.

By the end of my treatments, I was completely pain free, and have remained pain free for over a year and a half.

I am very happy at the outcome and would not hesitate to use this treatment again.

Sincerely
Patricia Van Witsen

1. Active Release Techniques LLC - Lower Extremity Manual.

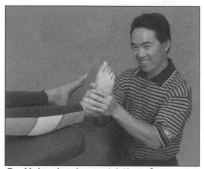

Dr. Mah releasing restrictions from the quadratus plantae and the flexor digitorum brevis.

By removing these soft-tissue restrictions, Active Release Techniques often achieves a functional resolution of this condition in a very short time period. It is not uncommon to see a significant reduction in symptoms in only 1 to 3 patient visits with resolution within 4 to 6 visits.

Once ART has been used to release the restrictions in these structures, the patient experiences an *immediate* change as the range of motion increases and the foot becomes less tender. In fact, patients are constantly amazed that, after only one treatment, they are able to stand comfortably on the foot, which only moments before, caused them excruciating pain.

Functional vs. Symptomatic Relief

The best treatment method should yield the best results. At our clinic, we aim to obtain the *permanent functional resolution* of the patient's Plantar Fasciitis. By this definition, a successful resolution of Plantar Fasciitis would be:

> '*A patient who returns to full work capacity with little or no discomfort, and who requires little or no maintenance treatment.'*

Compare this to a *symptomatic* solution, which simply aims to remove pain symptoms without actually resolving the problem.

A *functional* resolution aims to return the patient to their normal life activities, with little or no pain or discomfort.

100

Going the Extra Step - The Kinetic Chain

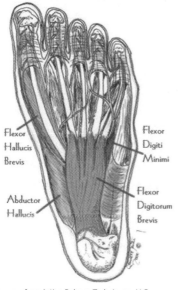
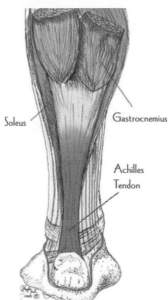

Images from Active Release Techniques, LLC

Research has shown that other structures, other than the plantar fascia and plantar aponeurosis, are involved in most cases of Plantar Fasciitis.[1] Other structures which cause, or are related to, excessive pronation include:

- Calf muscle restrictions in the gastrocnemius and soleus.
- Hamstring restrictions in the biceps femoris, semitendinosus, and semimembranosus muscles.
- Quadratus plantae, flexor digitorum brevis, flexor digiti minimi, abductor hallucis, and flexor hallucis brevis.

Further up the kinetic chain, structures such as the internal and external rotators of the hip can also cause problems with the biomechanics of the lower extremities. [2]

To ensure proper resolution of Plantar Fasciitis, ART practitioners always look beyond the immediate symptomatic area of the foot, and consider structures within the balance of the kinetic chain. By treating these additional soft-tissue structures, the practitioner is able to address the original biomechanical dysfunctions that may

1.   Kwong, P., Kay, D., & White, M. (1988). Plantar Fasciitis: Mechanics and pathomechanics of treatment. Clinical Sports Medicine, 7(1), 119-126
2.   Active Release Techniques LLC, Lower Extremity Manual., P. Michael Leahy, DC, CCSP, Copyright 2000

have caused the Plantar Fasciitis condition, and thereby prevent a reoccurrence of the problem.

Biomechanical analysis is also part of any ART analysis. During a biomechanical analysis, the practitioner:

- Identifies both the primary and antagonistic structures involved in the injury. The affected structures can vary greatly from individual to individual, although all patients may manifest the same physical pain symptoms.
- Locates the restrictive adhesions that have formed.
- Determines which other soft-tissue structures are affected along the structure's kinetic chain.

Active Release Techniques is successful at treating Plantar Fasciitis because it:

- Locates the unique, true, root cause of Plantar Fasciitis for each patient.
- Works along the entire kinetic chain – from the ankle, to the calf, the knee, the hamstrings, and into the hips – since the entire lower extremity may be involved and affected.
- Allows the practitioner to concurrently diagnose and treat. ART teaches that the best way to locate tissue restrictions is by *feeling* that restriction. This is where ART practitioners excel – with their superb sense of touch – and also where many other myofascial techniques (which may use hard metal, wooden, or plastic tools) fail.

ART is used to *find* the specific tissues that are restricted and to physically *work* them back to their normal texture, tension, and length, using various hand positioning and soft-tissue manipulation methods.

The actual sequence of treatments, and the sites addressed, vary depending on the individual, and the actual cause of the problem. All restrictions, along the entire kinetic chain, must be released to resolve the problem.

Why do Conventional Plantar Fasciitis Treatments Fail?

Conventional treatments for Plantar Fasciitis fail due to several factors:

- Treatments typically address just the plantar fascia, and do not address problems in other soft-tissues along the kinetic chain. This results in poor recovery, and future reoccurrences of the problem.
- Treatments often exacerbate the condition, rather than correct it.
- Treatments rarely affect the root cause of the problem.

Splints/braces

Splints increase, rather than decrease, the problems of Plantar Fasciitis because they:

- Restrict motion, thereby increasing stress further up the kinetic chain, resulting in yet more restrictions.
- Restrict circulation and flow of oxygen, causing production of new adhesions.
- Cause soft-tissues to atrophy and weaken when they are worn continuously.

Weakened tissues force other muscles to work harder, creating a biomechanical imbalance, with increasing friction, tension, and the continuation of the Cumulative Injury Cycle.

A Case History - Plantar Fasciitis

Sister Mary, a 72-year-old nun, is a classic example of how ART can help resolve Plantar Fasciitis. Sister Mary is a true caregiver. Each week she works hard and selflessly to provide care to seniors, many of whom are not much older than herself. She provides this care despite the excruciating pain she has experienced in her feet, every day, for the last twenty years.

Sister Mary initially came into our clinic seeking treatment for a severe case of Carpal Tunnel Syndrome (CTS). After resolving the CTS with ART, I suggested that we take a look at her feet and her Plantar Fasciitis problems.

Her initial reaction was to say "*That's okay dear, there's nothing you can do*". I insisted that we had a good chance at helping her. To this day, I am sure she only agreed in order to pacify and comfort me.

Upon examination, Sister Mary showed severe restrictions and adhesions in her feet, calf, hamstrings, and hips. The restrictions were so severe that it was almost miraculous that she was able to move as well as she did. After clearing these restrictions with only four ART treatments, Sister Mary found that she had *no pain* in either foot. I have never seen a nun this happy– she kept blessing me – over and over! Perhaps there's hope for me yet!

Plantar Fasciitis is an often poorly-treated condition which we are able to treat with consistently great results.

Exercises for Plantar Fasciitis

Once the restrictions and adhesed tissues have been released with ART, post-treatment exercises become a critical part of the healing process, and act to ensure the repetitive strain injury does not return. It is important to remember that exercises are only effective if they are executed *after* the adhesions within the soft-tissue have been released by ART treatments.

Attempts to stretch muscles that are currently bound by adhesions often do not achieve the desired results. In addition, only the muscles above and below the restrictions are lengthened. The actual restricted area remains unaffected, causing further muscle imbalances and stresses, and resulting in the formation of yet more restrictive tissues. This is why generic stretching exercises for Plantar Fasciitis seldom work.

In addition to stretching, a program of strengthening is also very important to ensure the problem does not return. The following pages depict some of the specific strengthening and stretching exercises that we recommend at our clinic for the prevention of Plantar Fasciitis.

- *Ankle Nerve Flossing - page 105.*
- *Arch Raise - page 105.*
- *Rolling Can - page 106.*
- *Stretching the Peroneals with a Wobble Board - page 106.*
- *Calf Stretch - Leaning Against Wall - page 107.*
- *Single Leg Stand - page 108.*

Ankle Nerve Flossing: This exercise stretches the nerves that pass through the ankle, and ensures they can translate smoothly through the surrounding soft-tissues.

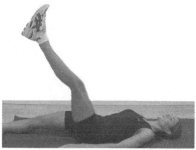 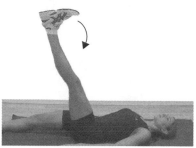

1. Lie on your back in a neutral position.

2. Lift up your affected leg so that your toes are pointing towards the ceiling. Your body should be relaxed with both hips in contact with the floor, and your affected leg slightly bent at the knee.

3. Slowly straighten your knee and simultaneously flex or pull your toes back
    towards the floor.

4. Repeat this exercise 10 times, for each leg.

Arch Raise : This exercise is designed to work the smaller, intrinsic muscles in the arch of your foot.

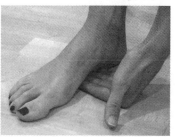 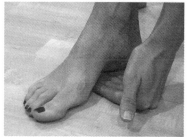

1. With your palm up, place the tips of your fingers under the arch of your foot

2. Move the arch of your foot away from your fingers, without crunching your toes in. This is a very subtle movement. It is important to keep the toes extended as you raise and lower the arch of your foot.

3. Raise the arch up for a count of one, hold up for 3 to 5 seconds, and then lower the arch back down.

4. Repeat this exercise 10 times for each foot.

Rolling Can: This exercise is especially effective when you get out of bed and find that your feet are too sensitive for walking. You will need a sturdy tin can, tennis ball, or bottle for this exercise.

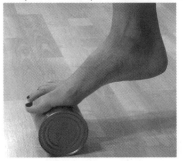 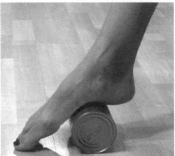

1.   Sit on a chair or on the side of your bed.

2.   Place your affected foot on the can.

3.   Gently roll the can back and forth under your foot. Roll from the balls of your feet to the back of the heel.

4.   Repeat this exercise 15 times without pausing.

5.   Repeat this exercise with the other foot.

Stretching the Peroneals with a Wobble Board: This exercise stretches the peroneal muscles which are very important for lateral stability of the ankle. You will need a wobble board for this exercise.

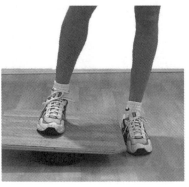 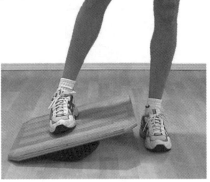

1.   Place your foot flat on the wobble board

2.   Allow the foot to invert (supinate). Hold this position for 30 seconds.

3.   Repeat this exercise with the other foot.

Calf Stretch - Leaning Against Wall: This two-part exercise stretches the gastrocnemius and soleus muscles.

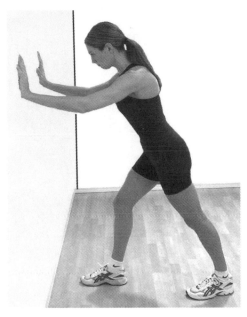

1. Face the wall and place the palms of your hands against the wall.

2. Move one leg back about 2 to 3 feet from the wall, making sure that both feet are facing directly forward, and the heel of the back foot remains firmly planted on the ground.

3. Lean forward towards the wall.

4. Now bend the front leg slightly, while keeping the back leg extended and straight. You should feel tension closer to the knee than to the ankle.

5. Hold this stretch for 30 seconds or until you feel a release of the tension.

6. Repeat this gastrocnemius stretch with the other leg.

7. Now, bring the back leg forward until there is a 6-inch gap between the two feet. Keep both feet pointing straight forward with heels firmly planted on the ground.

8. Bend both legs to create a stretch along the soleus muscles at the back of the lower legs. You should feel tension closer to the ankle than the knee for this stretch.

9. Hold this stretch for 30 seconds.

10. Repeat this exercise once for each side.

Single Leg Stand: This exercise increases your sense of balance, proprioception, and body awareness. You can start by standing, and progress to performing this exercise on a wobble board.

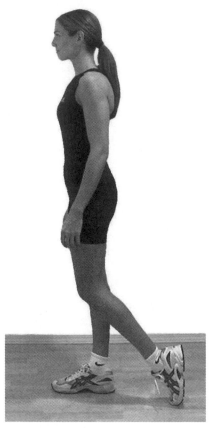
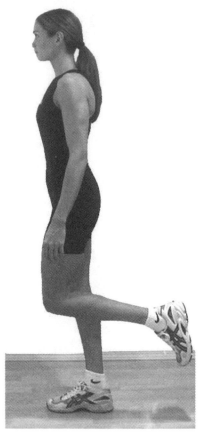

1. Stand in a relaxed position, hands at your side.

2. Slowly bend one leg until your foot is *off* the floor.

3. Balance on the other foot for 15 to 30 seconds.

4. Repeat with the other leg.

5. Repeat this exercise 3 times, for each leg.

6. Try the following variations once you are comfortable doing this exercise:
    - Balance with your eyes closed.
    - Balance on a wobble board – with your eyes *open*.

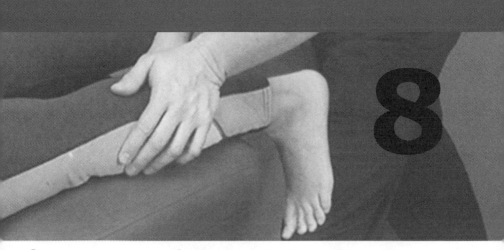

Injuries to the Achilles Tendon

In this chapter

Ask yourself:

- Does your Achilles tendon feel tender and swollen?
- Do you experience pain when you rise up on your toes?
- Do you have limited range of motion in your ankle?
- Do you experience pain with any action that stretches the Achilles tendon?

If you answered YES to one or more of the above questions, you may have Achilles Tendonitis or a related injury. These injuries are commonly diagnosed as paratenonitis, tendinosis, or rupture of the tendons. Most of these injuries can be effectively treated with Active Release Techniques (ART).

What Causes Injuries to the Achilles Tendon?

Injuries to the Achilles tendon are quite common and are often seen:

- In the weekend warrior who suddenly increases his or her physical activity, or suddenly starts a new sport without proper training, stretching, or preparation.
- In women who have changed from wearing high heels to low heels. In such situations, the Achilles tendon has become accustomed to remaining in a shortened position and is unable to adapt to the stretching required by wearing flat shoes.
- In athletes who suffer from overpronation, inflexibility, or lack of strength. Weakness in the gastrocnemius and soleus muscles can cause abnormal pronation during the stance phase of the normal gait cycle.[1]
- In runners who increase their mileage too rapidly, who attempt hill training without proper strengthening exercises, or who are using sub-standard running gear.
- In people with weak or unstable calf muscles, who suddenly place increased stress upon their Achilles tendon. A tight muscle is a weak muscle. Runners with weak or unstable calf muscles place increased stress upon their Achilles tendon.

The repetitive stresses caused by walking, running, cycling, or other sports can cause friction and inflammation in the area of the Achilles tendon. The body responds to this inflammation by laying down scar tissue (adhesive tissue) in an attempt to stabilize the area. Inflexibility is often caused by the build-up of these adhesions, either within the soft-tissue, or within structures above or below the tendon's kinetic chain.

Once this happens, an ongoing cycle begins that worsens the condition. For more information about this process, see:

- *The Cumulative Injury Cycle - page 12.*
- *Applying the Law of Repetitive Motion to CTS - page 43.*

---

1. Overuse Injuries in Ultraendurance Triathletes, American Journal of Sports Medicine, Vol. 17, pp. 514-518, 1989

About the Achilles Tendon

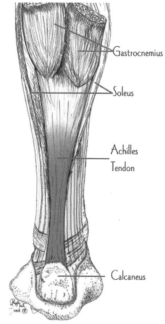

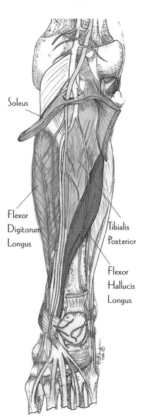

The Achilles tendon is the strongest and largest tendon in the body. It is extremely vulnerable to injury due to its limited blood supply and the numerous forces to which it is subjected.

The Achilles tendon is known as a co-joined tendon. This tendon joins directly into the calf muscles (gastrocnemius and soleus). The Achilles tendon transmits the force generated by the calf muscles to produce the push-off required for walking, running, and jumping.

Images from Active Release Techniques, LLC

The area of the Achilles tendon (approximately 2 to 6 cm above its insertion into the calcaneus) is very dense and under constant tension; consequently, this area has the poorest blood supply, which makes it extremely susceptible to injury and very slow to heal when it is injured.

The calf muscles associated with the Achilles tendon are composed of several layers of muscles, with the large gastrocnemius and soleus muscles being the more superficial. Under these muscles is a deeper layer of three muscles – the tibialis posterior, flexor hallucis longus, and flexor digitorum longus.

Injuries, restrictions, or adhesions in any of these tissue structures can directly affect the function and strength of the Achilles tendon.

Injuries to the Achilles Tendon

Injuries to the Achilles tendon can be caused by:

- Wearing shoes with high heels.
- Repetitive motions.
- Running up hills.
- Sudden increases in exercise routines.
- Tight or shortened calf muscles.
- Activities that require a sudden burst of speed.
- Jumping.

In our clinic, we commonly see three types of injuries to the Achilles tendon – paratenonitis, tendinosis, and rupture of the tendons:

Achilles Tendonitis/Paratenonitis: This injury is commonly known as Achilles Tendonitis and describes an inflammation of the *paratenon* - a sheath surrounding the Achilles tendon. Paratenonitis is often caused by overuse or repetitive strain and commonly occurs in triathletes and runners.

Tendinosis: Refers to degeneration within the Achilles tendon due to a previous tear. This condition can be felt as a palpable tendon nodule very close to the heel. The nodule is formed by the accumulation of scar tissue.

Circulation to the Achilles tendon is very poor, especially near the heel, resulting in poor oxygen supply. This results in poor healing and formation of microscopic tears, causing the tendon to thicken. Chronic Achilles Tendinosis can lead to a complete rupture of the tendon if it is not treated and rehabilitated correctly. If not addressed, this tendinosis may be a warning sign of worse things to come.

Rupture of the Tendon (either partial or complete): Refers to the tearing or separation of the *Achilles tendon* from the *calcaneus* (heel bone). The Achilles tendon is very strong and can withstand a force of 1000 pounds without tearing. However, even with this strength, the Achilles tendon is the second most frequently ruptured tendon in the body. A complete rupture is where the tendon has completely separated from the calcaneus (heel bone). This can occur when Paratenonitis and Tendinosis are not correctly treated and rehabilitated. Surgical intervention is the only solution for resolving a complete rupture of the Achilles tendon.

Conventional Treatments

We have seen numerous case of Achilles Tendonitis that were needlessly prolonged or that became chronic problems due to the application of ineffective treatments. Improper treatment of an Achilles Tendon injury can lead to major problems.

Many of our patients come to us after undergoing a series of ineffective treatments. In many cases these treatments often exacerbate or increase the amount of damage to the Achilles tendon. These include:

- The use of direct, heavy pressure and tension over the Achilles tendon.
- Cross-fiber massage which often irritates this area, increasing, rather than decreasing, the time required for recovery.
- Steroid injections, which should be avoided whenever possible. Research has shown that more than three or four steroid injections in a year can weaken tendons and damage joints, and can cause weight gain, diabetes, osteoporosis, and ulcers. [1]

Treating the Achilles Tendon with ART

Active Release Techniques is very successful at treating injuries of the Achilles tendon, as it addresses the release of restrictive adhesions between both superficial and deep tissue structures – not just at the Achilles tendon, but also all along the soft-tissue structures of its kinetic chain.

The Need for a Specific Diagnosis

It is extremely important to be as specific as possible when identifying the soft-tissue structures involved with Achilles Tendonitis. Patients may present with identical pain patterns at the Achilles tendon, yet have completely different structures that are impairing motion or causing the injury.

---

1. *A Different Look at Corticosteroids*, ROGER J. ZOOROB, M.D., M.P.H., Louisiana State University Medical Center, DAWN CENDER, PHARM.D.,University of Kentucky A.B. Chandler Medical Center, Lexington, Kentucky, American Family Physician, August 1998

Before treatment takes place, we perform a very specific examination and diagnosis of the Achilles tendon and its related structures. It is important to look past the initial point of pain and identify all the other structures that are involved in the kinetic chain.

For example, if the fascial tissue anterior to the tendon is restricted (which commonly occurs in injuries to the Achilles tendon), ART protocols can be followed for releasing these adhesions, without placing stress on the tendon itself.

Structures of the Achilles Tendon's Kinetic Chain

Other structures of the Achilles tendon's kinetic chain that we commonly find in cases of Achilles tendon injuries include:

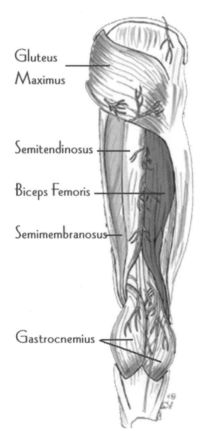

Gluteus
Maximus

Semitendinosus

Biceps Femoris

Semimembranosus

Gastrocnemius

Images from Active Release Techniques, LLC

- The hamstrings, which is a group of muscles which includes the biceps femoris, semitendinosus, and semimembranosus. Tension in these muscles causes more stress upon the muscles of the lower leg.

- The tibialis posterior, which lies deep to the calf muscles. This muscle inverts the foot, (turns the foot inwards) and plantar flexes the foot (helps you to point your toes down).

- The popliteus muscle, which lies deep behind the knee and is involved in medial knee rotation. When it is restricted, it may place increased stress upon the lower extremities.

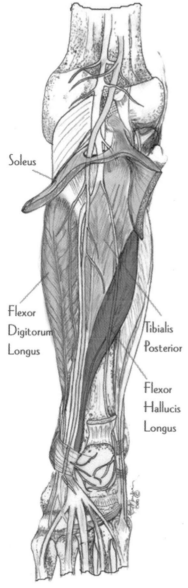

Soleus

Flexor
Digitorum
Longus

Tibialis
Posterior

Flexor
Hallucis
Longus

Images from Active Release Techniques, LLC

- The soleus muscle, which is a powerful plantar flexor of the foot and gives you the ability to rise up on your toes.

- The flexor digitorum longus works to flex toes 2 thru 5. It also helps to plantar flex the foot.

- The flexor hallucis longus, flexor hallucis brevis, and the tibialis anterior muscles, which are all involved in cases of increased pronation and hyperpronation.

- The plantaris muscle, which inserts into the middle one third of the posterior calcaneal surface (heel bone), just on the inside of the Achilles tendon. This muscle assists in plantar flexion of the foot and is also involved in flexion of the leg.

Since ART protocols are structure-specific and based upon the individual needs of each athlete, the practitioner is able to customize each treatment to include the specific soft-tissue structures involved in the injury.

Each Achilles tendon injury is treated as a unique case, with treatments being applied to only those structures that require attention.

A Case History - Achilles Tendon

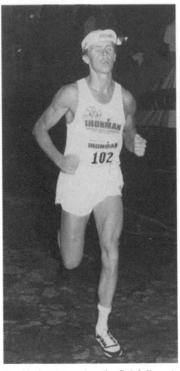

Dr. Abelson crossing the finish line at 1982 Kona Ironman Championships.

I have been a marathon runner involved in the local running community for the last twenty years. With this running came a wide variety of personal injuries. I always joke about how I only get injuries so that I can learn about how to effectively treat them.

Many years ago, I had this brilliant idea that if we started doing more of our long training runs on mountain trails, we would improve our running times. Within a very short period of time most of my running group started to have problems with their Achilles tendons. To say the least, they were not very happy with me.

I ended up injuring my own Achilles tendon so badly that I had to drop out of a race for which I had trained for six months. In fact, it took about *three months of therapy* before I could even attempt running again.

Today, I try to keep those brilliant ideas to myself, and have learned much quicker, and more effective ways for treating this painful condition.

On a more recent and positive note, I would like to tell you about one my patients, June. June is a natural runner! In her first year of running she started with only a few short runs per week. By the end of the year she had qualified for the Boston Marathon with a time of 3:20 at her first local marathon.

Unfortunately, June had not built a sufficient running base to allow her to withstand the stresses she was placing on her body. She came into my office with an injury to her Achilles tendon just two weeks before the Boston Marathon.

June was literally limping down the hall saying, '*Fix me, I need to run the Boston Marathon in two weeks.*' I didn't want to get her hopes up too high since I only had two weeks within which to achieve her treatment goals. However, June told me that she was going to run the race, no matter what!

Unlike many people who suffer from injuries to the Achilles tendon, June was not a heavy pronator. Her physical examination showed that she had not been focusing on her stretching. Everything was tight, from her ankles, up through her calfs, hamstrings, gluteals, and even her lower back. The same level of tightness appeared on the non-injured side as well, indicating high stress on that side too, with a good chance that her other leg could soon see a similar injury. The most prevalent restrictions were found in her calf muscles and hamstrings.

The calf muscles are composed of several layers of muscles, with the large gastrocnemius and soleus muscles being the more superficial. Under these there is a deeper layer containing three muscles called the tibialis posterior, flexor hallucis longus, and flexor digitorum longus. I noticed on examination that the relative translation and movement of these structures was extremely limited.

I had to perform several ART procedures on June's calf muscles and hamstrings before anything began to loosen. There was very little change in function that first day, but there was some pain relief. In fact, June's muscles were so tight and restricted, that it was not until her 4th visit that I actually felt the release in the tissues that I needed to feel.

At that time, I asked June to walk up and down the hall again. There was a definite improvement this time. I told her to try running in a few days. June, a very motivated individual, was more than willing to give it a try.

I didn't get to see June again for almost a month. When June finally did come in, it was not for her injury, but to show me her pictures of the Boston Marathon. She couldn't have been happier! She had run a great race with absolutely no pain!

Obviously most of my patients who have problems with their Achilles tendon are not a few weeks away from running the Boston Marathon. But they are frequently able to achieve the same kind of positive results with ART treatments.

Exercises for Achilles Tendon Injuries

Once the restrictions and adhesed tissues have been released with ART, post-treatment exercises become a critical part of the healing process, and act to ensure the repetitive strain injury does not return.

It is important to remember that exercises are only effective if they are executed *after* the adhesions within the soft-tissue have been released by ART treatments.

Attempts to stretch muscles that are currently bound by adhesions often do not achieve the desired results. In addition, only the muscles above and below the restrictions are lengthened. The actual restricted area remains unaffected, causing further muscle imbalances and stresses, and resulting in the formation of yet more restrictive tissues. This is why generic stretching exercises for Achilles Tendonitis seldom work.

In addition to stretching, a program of strengthening is also very important to ensure the problem does not return. The following pages depict some of the specific strengthening and stretching exercises that we recommend at our clinic for the prevention of Achilles Tendonitis.

- *Calf Stretch - Leaning Against Wall - page 119.*
- *Single Leg Hamstring Stretch - page 120.*
- *Unilateral Partial Squat - page 121.*
- *Single Leg Stand - page 122.*
- *Single Leg Lunge on a SitFitter® - page 123.*

Calf Stretch - Leaning Against Wall: This two-part exercise stretches both the gastrocnemius and soleus muscles.

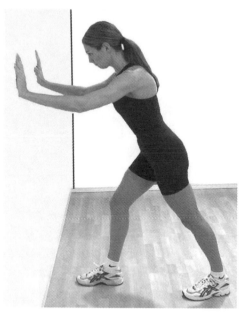

1. Face the wall and place the palms of your hands against the wall.

2. Move one leg back about 2 to 3 feet, making sure that both feet are facing directly forward, and the heel of your back foot remains firmly planted on the ground.

3. Lean forward towards the wall.

4. Now bend the front leg slightly, while keeping the back leg extended and straight. You should feel tension closer to the knee than to the ankle.

5. Hold this stretch for 30 seconds or until you feel a release of the tension.

6. Repeat this gastrocnemius stretch with the other leg.

7. Now, bring the back leg forward until there is a 6 inch gap between the two feet. Keep both feet pointing straight forward with heels firmly planted on the ground.

8. Bend both legs to create a stretch along the soleus muscles at the back of the lower legs. You should feel tension closer to the ankle than to the knee for this stretch.

9. Hold this stretch for 30 seconds.

10. Repeat this exercise once for each side.

Single Leg Hamstring Stretch: This exercise stretches and increases the flexibility of the gluteal fold, hamstrings, and calf muscles of the affected leg.

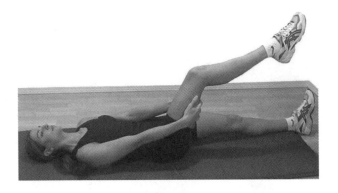

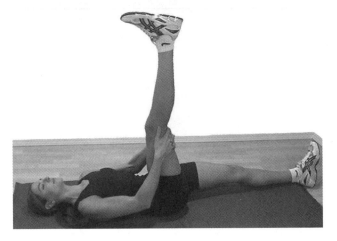

1. Lie on your back.
2. With both hands, reach down and clasp your leg just above the knee.
3. Lift the leg up towards the ceiling and pull the leg towards your chest, keeping the leg straight throughout the motion.
   - Only stretch to the point where you feel a light tension on the back of your leg. Do not overstretch.
   - You may feel the tension in the upper or lower portion of the leg.
   - Normal range of motion is about 80 to 90 degrees as measured from the floor.
4. Hold the stretch for 30 seconds and repeat it for the other side.

Unilateral Partial Squat: This strengthening exercise combines proprioception and balance to train the gluteal muscles to work in coordination with the muscles of the thigh. Make sure you keep your hip, knee, and second toe of the standing leg vertically aligned over each other as you do this exercise.

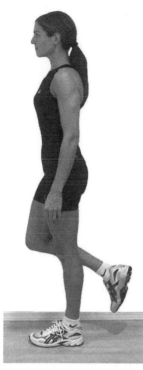

1. Stand sideways to the wall, with your shoulder about 3 to 4 inches from the wall.

    If necessary, you can also lean lightly against the wall, for additional support.

2. Bend the leg of the inner foot, while balancing on the outer foot.

3. Slowly squat down as far you can while maintaining your alignment and balance.

    Ensure that the leg closest to the wall remains parallel to the wall throughout the exercise.

4. Come back up at the same speed.

5. Repeat this exercise 12 to 20 times for each side.

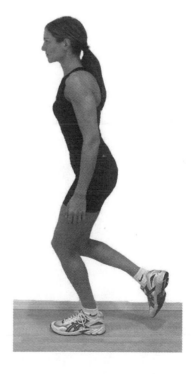

Single Leg Stand: This exercise increases your sense of balance, proprioception, and body awareness. You can start by standing, and progress to performing this exercise on a wobble board.

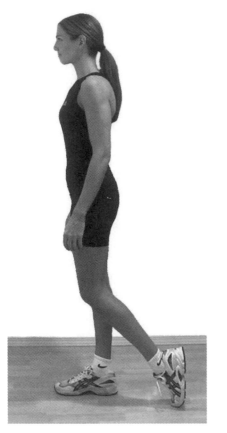
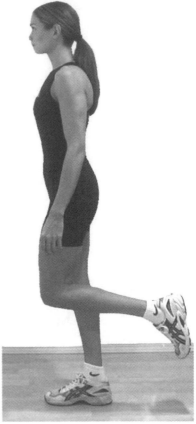

1. Stand in a relaxed position, hands at your side.

2. Slowly bend one leg until your foot is *off* the floor.

3. Balance on the other foot for 15 to 30 seconds.

4. Repeat with the other leg.

5. Repeat this exercise 3 times, for each leg.

6. Try the following variations once you are comfortable doing this exercise:
   - Balance with your eyes closed.
   - Balance on a wobble board – with your eyes *open*.

Single Leg Lunge on a SitFitter®: You will need to use a SitFitter for this exercise. This exercise stimulates and strengthens the muscles surrounding the hip, ankle, and knee. This is an advanced exercise that should only be done after you are comfortable with the Unilateral Partial Squat (see page 121).

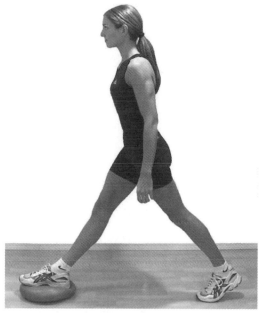

1. Place one foot flat on the Sit-Fitter. Place the other leg as far back as you comfortably can.

2. Drop the back knee to the floor while keeping the front foot flat on the SitFitter. Ensure your posture is upright throughout the movement and that your front leg is doing all of the work. Do not allow the knee to extend beyond the front of the foot.

3. Go up and down 12 to 20 times for each side.

4. Repeat for the other side for the *same* number of repetitions.

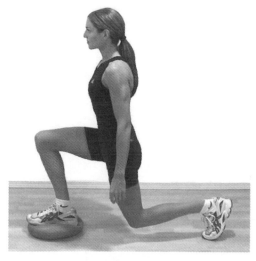

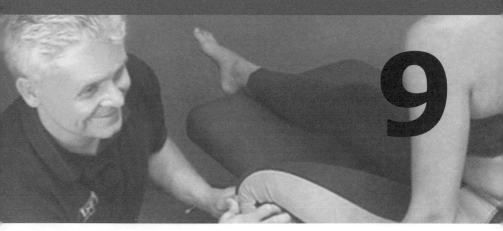

Knee Injuries

Ask yourself:

- Do you experience pain on the outer or inner sides of your knees?
- Do you experience pain above, below, or under your knee cap?
- Do you experience pain in your knees while walking, running, or jumping?
- Do you experience pain in your knees while getting up from a chair or while going up or down stairs?
- Do you experience pain in your knees when driving or sitting for extended periods of time?

If you answered YES to one or more of the above questions, you may have a knee problem that can be helped with Active Release Techniques.

What Causes Knee Pain

As a runner and a sports medicine practitioner, I commonly see people with a variety of knee injuries. The causes of the knee pain are varied and often result from a combination of environmental, physical, and physiological factors. Knee pain can be caused by:

- Repetitive motion injuries.
- Muscle imbalances.
- Osteoarthritis.
- Tendonitis.
- Ligament injury.
- Meniscus injuries.
- Iliotibial Band Syndrome.
- Osgood-Schlatter Disease.
- A variety of pathological processes. Pathological causes of knee pain are rare compared to the more common mechanical causes of knee pain.

These conditions, if left untreated, can often lead to an ongoing cycle of biomechanical imbalances which eventually lead to ongoing pain and degeneration of the knee, as well as hip, low back, shoulder, or neck problems. Our body is composed of a series of structural kinetic chains, where a dysfunction or imbalance in one area can quickly lead to dysfunctions in other parts of the body.

Sometimes surgery is necessary to correct knee problems, but in the majority of cases it is not. By applying the right treatment procedures and proper rehabilitative programs, most people can not only treat their current knee problem, but can also prevent future knee injuries from occurring.

About Your Knee

The knee is a complex structure made up of bones, joints, muscles, ligaments, tendons, and cartilage. The knee plays a vital role in all gait-related tasks and its function is greatly affected by the condition of soft-tissue structures both above and below the knee. Many treatment methods fail to fully resolve knee injuries since they do not address the complex and varying interrelationships between the various soft-tissue structures that make up the knee.

Bones of the Knee

The knee is a hinge joint consisting of the following three bones and the knee cap or patella:

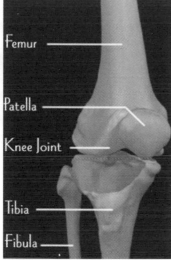

Femur

Patella

Knee Joint

Tibia

Fibula

Image courtesy of Primal Pictures Ltd.
www.anatomy.tv

- The femur is a large bone in the thigh that extends from your hip joint to the knee. The quadriceps muscles attach to this bone.
- The tibia (or shin bone) is the larger of the two bones, which extends from your knee to your foot.
- The fibula is the smaller of the two bones, which extends from the outside of your knee to your foot. It lies on the outside (lateral side) of the tibia.

The patella (or knee cap) is a sesamoid bone – a bone that is covered by a ligament or tendon. The patella lies under the quadriceps tendon and functions as a fulcrum to increase the strength of the quadriceps muscles. The patella is held in place by the quadriceps tendon above, and the patellar ligament underneath. Additional thin ligaments on the outer and inner sides also help to hold the patella in place. See the image – *page 129* for more details.

Ligaments of the Knee

A ligament is a tough band of white, fibrous, slightly elastic tissue that forms an essential part of skeletal joints, and acts to bind bones together. Ligaments prevent dislocation, and restrict excessive movement that might cause injury.

There are four main ligaments as well as a ligamentous structure that should be considered for all knee problems.

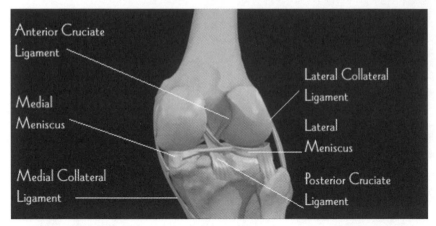

Anterior Cruciate Ligament

Medial Meniscus

Medial Collateral Ligament

Lateral Collateral Ligament

Lateral Meniscus

Posterior Cruciate Ligament

Image courtesy of Primal Pictures Ltd.
www.anatomy.tv

- The Iliotibial Band (ITB), is a wide, flat, ligamentous structure that originates at the iliac crest and inserts onto the outer aspect of the tibia, just below the knee. The ITB serves as a ligamentous connection between the femur (at the lateral femoral epicondyle) and the lateral tibia (at Gerdy's Tubercle). The ITB is not attached to bone as it passes between the femur and the tibia. This allows the ITB to move forward and backward with knee flexion and extension. See the illustration – *page 129* for more details.
- The Anterior Cruciate Ligament (ACL), which is located in the center of the knee, limits the rotation and forward movement of the tibia.
- The Posterior Cruciate Ligament (PCL), which is located in the center of the knee, limits backward movement of the tibia.
- The Medial Collateral Ligament (MCL) provides stability to the inner area of the knee.
- The Lateral Collateral Ligament (LCL) provides stability to the outer area of the knee.

Meniscus

The meniscus is a circular-shaped cartilage in your knees that acts as a shock absorber, helping to spread out the weight being transferred during gait from the femur to the tibia. There are two menisci in each knee, the lateral meniscus and the medial meniscus.

The ability of the meniscus to spread out these forces is very important since, in doing so, it helps to protect the articular cartilage of the knee. Articular cartilage allows smooth articulation of joint surfaces and cushions the forces exerted on the knees.

Since the bottom of the femur is round, and the top of the tibia is flat, the meniscus also allows these two differently-shaped surfaces to slide smoothly over one another.

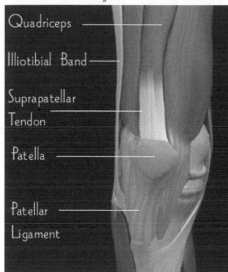

Quadriceps

Illiotibial Band

Suprapatellar
Tendon

Patella

Patellar
Ligament

Image courtesy of Primal Pictures Ltd.
www.anatomy.tv

Tendons

Tendons are extremely strong cords of connective tissue that connect muscle to bone, and are the termination point for muscles.

The quadriceps muscles (at the front of your thigh) connect to the patella (knee cap) via the supra-patellar tendon.

The patella connects to the tibia via the infra-patellar tendon.

Muscles and the Kinetic Chain Relationships

When dealing with any knee injury, your practitioner should consider all the anatomical structures both above and below the knee. New patterns of dysfunction will develop whenever any segment of the knee's kinetic chain is not functioning properly.

Common muscular structures above and below the knee that must be considered for any knee injury include:

- Hip extensors.
- Hip flexors.

- Internal and external hip rotators.
- Calf muscles.
- Structures below the knee in lateral, medial, anterior, and posterior directions.
- Structures involved in normal ankle and foot motion.

For an example of the importance of the knee's kinetic chain, let us take a look at a person whose foot is *excessively pronated* (rolled inwards). This pronation causes the person's foot to flatten out during normal walking. This flattening then causes the tibia to rotate inwards (medially) and the femur to rotate outward (laterally). These actions place a considerable amount of stress on the knee, eventually leading to friction, inflammation, and injury of the soft-tissues of the knee. Thus, a problem that started at the foot ends up causing abnormal hip and femur rotation, which in turn leads to knee problems.

It is possible to achieve moderate success by treating just the immediate structures of the knee. However, in order to truly resolve the problem, we should also treat those structures that were the *original* cause of the excessive pronation – that is, the structures in the knee's kinetic chain. For example, restriction in any of the following structures may be the cause of the excessive pronation:

- Peroneus longus and peroneus brevis muscles are responsible for allowing you to point your feet and for eversion (rolling inward) of the foot when walking or running.
- Abductor hallucis is responsible for flexing the big toe and allows your big toe to move laterally (sideways). This is important since the normal walking/running stride requires us to push-off with our big toe.
- Flexor hallucis brevis is responsible for flexing the big toe and for supporting the medial arch of the foot.
- Tibialis anterior lets you bend your foot upwards (dorsiflexion) and also helps to invert the foot (roll outwards) when you walk. The inversion of the foot is an important part of the normal gait pattern.
- Flexor hallucis longus is responsible for flexing the big toe, supinating the ankle (turning inwards), and in pointing your foot (plantar flexion).

Restrictions in any of these structures can cause pronation, which in turn leads to hip restrictions, and subsequent knee problems. Obviously, in such situations, treating just the structures of the knee will *not* resolve the knee problem. Instead, the practitioner must treat the knee, and then, based on the biomechanical and ART analysis, treat all other affected structures in the knee's kinetic chain. The knee problem will only be resolved when restrictions in *all* these affected structures are removed. ART practitioners should perform a similar kinetic chain analysis for each and every dysfunction that they encounter.

Diagnostic Tools for the Knee

Doctors use a wide variety of methods to diagnose knee problems. Each of these diagnostic tools provide valuable information but each has its own limitations. A better approach would be to combine the results of these standard tools with the results obtained from a careful and complete biomechanical analysis and evaluation of soft-tissue translation.

Both traditional and conservative treatments use similar diagnostic tools to obtain information about the current condition of the knees. These tools include:

History - Your practitioner should ask you for a detailed and complete injury history. This fundamental component often provides more of a clue to the real problem than the most expensive diagnostic tools.

Physical examination - Traditionally a good physical knee examination should cover inspection, palpation, ranges of motion, circulatory, orthopedic, and neurological tests. In addition, an often missed step is a complete biomechanical assessment that checks the function of structures through the complete kinetic chain of the knee, from the hips right down to the feet.

X-rays - X-rays are valuable tools for ruling out a suspected fracture or other pathology. Just remember that X-rays tell you very little, or nothing, about soft-tissue damage. Since most knee injuries are due to soft-tissue problems, X-rays often provide little value other than for ruling out the existence of pathological conditions. See *The value of X-rays for pain diagnosis - page 174* for more information about X-rays.

CAT (Computerized Axial Tomography) Scans - CAT Scans can produce a series of cross-sectional images of the knee. CAT Scan images show soft-tissues more clearly than normal X-rays; however, it is very important to ensure that the practitioner has correlated these images to the symptom patterns and physical findings reported by the patient.

MRI (Magnetic resonance imaging) - MRI uses magnetic energy to produce signals that are detected by a scanner and then analyzed and interpreted by a computer. MRI technology is very good for detecting damage to soft-tissues.

But again, MRIs are nothing more than a good picture, unless the practitioner correlates these images to the symptom patterns and physical findings. By mapping the results of the MRI to symptom patterns, and to the results of a good physical examination, the practitioner can develop an effective roadmap for the treatment of knee injuries.

Biomechanical Analysis and the Kinetic Chain - This important diagnostic step is often missed, or, when performed, is conducted at a superficial and ineffective level.

An analysis of the knee's entire kinetic chain (both above and below the injury) must be performed in order to identify all the structures that are involved in causing this injury. This is the only way to ensure that a complete and effective treatment plan has been implemented. New dysfunctions of the knee and its related structures will continue to occur unless all the soft-tissue structures in the kinetic chain are treated and restored to proper working order.

Traditional Treatments and Perspectives

Knee pain can be caused by trauma, repetitive motion, or inflammation of any of the soft-tissue structures that either make up the knee, or that are associated with the knee's kinetic chain. See the following for a description of some typical knee problems:

- *Tendonitis/Tendinosis - page 133.*
- *Ligamentous Injury - page 133.*
- *Arthritis - page 134.*
- *Chondromalacia - page 136.*

Tendonitis/Tendinosis - Tendonitis refers to inflammation of a tendon. Tendonitis in the knee is commonly caused by activities that shorten the quadriceps, and that transfer force directly to the tendons of the knee. This force causes friction and inflammation of the tendons.

Tendonitis of the knee is common in ball players, runners, cyclists and triathletes. It is also common in the elderly, or in very inactive individuals. Untreated tendonitis can eventually lead to tearing and rupture of the tendon.

Traditionally, tendonitis/tendinosis is usually treated by icing during the acute stages of the injury, by reducing physical activities, and by the consumption of non-steroidal anti-inflammatory drugs (NSAIDs). These are short-term treatments that should only be applied during the acute stages of the injury. Most of these treatments are limited in their effects, and they provide only symptomatic relief – they act to reduce inflammation – but do not address the underlying biomechanical problems causing tendonitis/tendinosis.

In addition, the long-term consumption of non-steroidal anti-inflammatory medications has several detrimental side-effects including gastrointestinal problems, ulcerations, and internal bleeding. See *The effectiveness of pain medications* - *page 176* for more information.

See *ART and Tendonitis/Tendinosis* - *page 139* to learn how ART treats this condition.

Ligamentous Injury - There are four main ligaments in the knee which can be injured.

- Anterior cruciate ligament (ACL) is often injured by a sudden rotational motion of the knee.

- Posterior cruciate ligament (PCL) is often injured by the effects of a direct impact such as might occur in a sporting event, or a motor vehicle impact.

- Medial collateral ligament (MCL) is often injured by some type of trauma to the outside of the knee. MCL injuries are common in hockey, football, rugby, or other high-contact sports.

- Lateral collateral ligament (LCL) can be injured by an impact to the inside of the knee.

See the diagram – *page 128* for more information about this structure.

The types of traditional treatments prescribed for ligamentous injuries is dependent upon the degree of injury and the type of activities the patient will be involved in after the injury. Ligamentous injuries are classified into the following major grades:

- Grade 1 describes microscopic tears of the ligament.
- Grade 2 describes partial tears of the ligament.
- Grade 3 describes complete tears or rupture of the ligament.

Grade 1 injuries typically respond well to soft-tissue treatments and rehabilitative therapies. Grade 2 injuries also respond well to soft-tissue treatments, and generally do not require surgical intervention if treated correctly. Grade 3 injuries require surgical intervention to correct the problem.

See *ART and Ligament and Meniscus Injuries - page 140* to learn how ART treats this condition.

Arthritis - Osteoarthritis is the most common form of arthritis of the knee. This is a degenerative condition where the articular (surrounding) cartilage of the knee joint gradually breaks down. Osteoarthritis of the knee is characterized by:

- Morning stiffness.
- Swelling.
- Pain.
- Decreased range of motion.

Articular cartilage of the knee is quite different from other soft-tissue structures since it does not receive nourishment directly from the arterial blood flow. Instead the articular cartilage of the knee is completely dependent upon the pumping actions generated by physical movement to supply its nourishment. As you move, the ligaments and tendons surrounding the knee joint work to pump nutrients and blood (oxygen) to the cartilage of the knee.

Degeneration of the cartilage starts to occur when anything disrupts this flow.

Internal pressure within muscles, ligaments, or tendons creates a compressive stress that inhibits the flow of blood to the cartilage. This decreases the amount of oxygen that is getting to the cartilage, resulting in several enzymatic changes. These changes cause degeneration of the cartilage, with the upshot being an acceleration of the arthritic process.[1]

Repetitive strain is one of the key causes of osteoarthritis. Other factors that can stress soft-tissues or exacerbate this condition include muscle imbalances, biomechanical imbalances, excessive weight gain, a history of trauma, and hypoxia (lack of oxygen to inflamed tissues).

When an individual develops osteoarthritis, they show a corresponding decrease in the range-of-motion of the affected joint. This restriction in motion causes muscles to weaken and become shortened, fibrotic, and less flexible. Consequently, the muscles can no longer act as shock absorbers for the joints that they surround. This causes an increase in the amount of force being transferred to the joint. Eventually these stresses cause friction, inflammation, and an ongoing cycle of repetitive injury.

By using ART to release the restrictions in the surrounding soft-tissues, we can restore the flow of blood to the cartilage, thereby increasing oxygen levels for the tissues, and accelerating the body's healing process.

Recently, a great deal of controversy has arisen about the validity and effectiveness of many conventional procedures (surgical procedures, anti-inflammatory medications, and steroidal injections) that are used to treat osteoarthritis (OA) of the knee.

For example, every year an estimated 650,000 arthroscopic procedures are performed, costing over $3.5 billion dollars. *Knee surgery is big business!* Yet a recent study in the New England Journal of Medicine found this procedure was no better than a placebo[2]. This study clearly calls into question the legitimacy of this expensive and invasive procedure.

1.   Mapp, P.I., Grootveld, M.C., et al. 'Hypoxia, oxidative stress and rheumatoid arthritis.' Br Med Bull, 51(2): 419-436, 1995.
2.   JB Moseley et al. A controlled trial of arthroscopic surgery for Osteoarthritis of the knee. New England Journal of Medicine 2002 347: 81-88.

There is another consequence to these invasive surgical procedures. When cartilage is removed from the knee, the knee becomes very susceptible to further damage. The remaining cartilage begins to wear down. Once the cartilage wears out completely, you are left with *bone rubbing on bone*. Performing the first surgery simply hastens the likelihood of future knee replacement surgeries.

We strongly recommend that patients first research and attempt alternatives to surgical resolution of arthritis of the knee.

■ See *Is surgery really required? - page 177* for more information.
■ See *ART and Osteoarthritis of the Knee - page 141* to learn how ART treats this condition.

Chondromalacia - This condition is characterized by degeneration of the cartilage on the undersurface of the kneecap and can manifest as:

■ Pain on the sides of the knees or beneath the knee caps.
■ Occasional grinding sounds as you walk down the stairs.

Chondromalacia can be caused by muscle imbalances in the anterior and posterior muscles of the legs or by imbalances in gait such as excessive pronation or supination. See *ART and Chondromalacia - page 141* to learn how ART treats this condition.

Iliotibial Band Syndrome (ITBS) or Runner's Knee - This condition frequently occurs in long distance runners, sprinters, cyclists, and triathletes. ITBS presents as a sharp or burning pain on the lateral aspect of the knee. It can also cause pain to radiate up the side of the hip or thigh.

ITBS is an overuse injury caused by the repetitive action of the iliotibial band (ITB):

■ As it moves across the lateral femoral epicondyle. See *page 128* and *page 129* for more information about the iliotibial band.
■ When the knee is flexed at an angle greater than 30 degrees, and the iliotibial band moves back behind the lateral femoral epicondyle.
■ During knee extension, when the iliotibial band shifts forward in front of the lateral femoral epicondyle.

When the ITB is shortened or stressed, the repetitive actions of the knee during running and walking cause friction and inflammation of the iliotibial band. With ITBS, the bursa often becomes inflamed, manifesting as a clicking sensation as the knee flexes and extends.

RICE (Rest, Ice, Compression, Elevation) is usually recommended during the acute phases of the injury. This treatment is often combined with stretching of the hamstrings, gluteal musculature, and hip adductors. In addition, non-steroidal anti-inflammatory drugs (NSAIDs) are often prescribed to control pain and inflammation. See *The effectiveness of pain medications - page 176* for more information.

All these treatments provide symptomatic relief; they are treatments that take away or hide the signs or signals of the problem. These symptomatic treatments alleviate the patient's perception of pain, without dealing with the underlying cause of the problem. For example, medication provides symptomatic relief by *hiding* the pain signals generated by a broken leg, but it does not fix the broken leg.

Again, these conventional procedures *do* help during the acute stage by providing symptomatic relief, but they do *not* address or treat the true underlying biomechanical dysfunction.

See *ART and Iliotibial Band Syndrome (ITBS or Runner's Knee) - page 142* to learn how ART treats this condition.

RICE is always a good idea during the acute stages of *any* injury. And no...we are not talking about the jasmine or basmati varieties!

- **R for Rest** to slow down bleeding and reduce the risk of further injury. Only rest for short periods of time since too much rest can cause other problems.

- **I for Ice** to decrease pain, reduce swelling, reduce bleeding, and encourage circulation. Apply ice to the injured area for 15 to 20 minutes or until just numb. Do *not* use heat while the swelling is present since heat on an injured area will increase the swelling.

- **C for Compression** to reduce bleeding and swelling.

- **E for Elevation** to reduce bleeding and swelling by using the *positive* effects of gravity.

Meniscus Injuries - The menisci are commonly injured by repetitive actions or by an impact that also involves rotation of the knee. Meniscus injuries are characterized by swelling, clicking, or even locking of the knee in severe cases.

As with other types of cartilage, the menisci have a very poor blood supply, so anything that reduces the motion and replacement of the fluid around the knee will reduce healing.

Traditional treatments typically recommend surgery for a meniscus tear, especially if the damage is severe or when the injury is interfering with a person's ability to perform their normal daily activities.   However, it is important to remember that a tear in the meniscus does *not* mean you must have surgery. The need for surgery is dependent upon the severity of the tear. Many patients are able to function quite well despite a tear in the meniscus.

The two most commonly recommended surgical options for menisci are:

■   An attempt to *repair* the meniscus. This method has a better prognosis (outcome) but requires a longer time for recovery.

■   Performance of a menisectomy where a part of the meniscus is removed. This method has a fast recovery but can result in long-term complications.

See *ART and Ligament and Meniscus Injuries - page 140* to learn how ART treats this condition.

Osgood-Schlatter Disease - This condition is most commonly seen in athletic boys ranging in age from 9 to13 years of age. Osgood-Schlatter Disease is often experienced by individuals participating in activities that require jumping, running, or stair climbing. It's commonly seen in soccer, football, and basketball players.

This condition manifests as pain just below the knee – in the tibial tuberosity (upper part of tibia). Osgood-Schlatter Disease is caused by a chronic shortening of the quadriceps. The quadriceps connect to the patellar ligament. The ligament runs through the knee and into the tibia. When the quadriceps contract during activity, the patellar ligament pulls away from the tibia, causing pain. In time, a bump may appear where the ligament is being pulled away from the bone.

Traditional treatments typically include advice to the patient to stop all physical activities – that is, stop running, stop playing baseball, soccer, or any other sport. In addition, physicians often suggest

RICE (Rest, Ice, Compression, and Elevation) to be used in conjunction with stretching and strengthening exercises.

If this doesn't work, the physician may suggest the use of some sort of support, brace, or even crutches with the idea of reducing tension on the knee tendons and quadriceps muscles. As a last resort, surgery may be suggested. (I have never seen a case of Osgood-Schlatter Disease that required surgery to resolve this condition.)

See *ART and Osgood-Schlatter Disease - page 143* to learn how ART treats this condition.

ART and the Treatment of Knee Pain

I believe that the ART focus upon the restoration of normal translation and movement to all the soft-tissues that make up the knee's kinetic chain is the key to treating any soft-tissue-related knee condition. By using the ART methodology, we not only treat the current problem, but we can also help the patient prevent further knee injuries, and improve the patient's overall physical performance.

I have been very pleased with Active Release Techniques as it allows me to find the restricted areas, and then provides a means to remove these restrictions, thereby treating all the affected soft-tissue structures of the knee's kinetic chain. By doing this, we have obtained excellent resolution for all but the most critical forms of knee injuries.

ART and Tendonitis/Tendinosis - The suffix "itis" means inflammation. This can be quite misleading since a tendon injury, by itself, does not cause swelling or inflammation. We have found that swelling and inflammation at the knee usually indicates an accompanying ligamentous injury (medial or lateral meniscus) or a joint capsule problem.

The initial diagnosis of Tendonitis/Tendinosis often requires the treatment and removal of soft-tissue restrictions from not just the tendons, but also from other soft-tissue structures associated with the tendon's kinetic chain. These can include ligaments, muscles, knee joint capsule, neurological structures, and vascular structures.

In fact, with a typical ART treatment for Tendonitis/Tendinosis, we often find and remove restrictions in structures above, below, inside, and outside the actual tendons of the knee. By doing this, we are able to restore full function to the tendons, ligaments, muscles, knee joint capsule, and neurological and vascular structures that may have been the original cause of the tendonitis.

ART and Ligament and Meniscus Injuries - The type of treatment that I recommend for a ligamentous or meniscus injury is dependent upon the severity and extent of the injury.

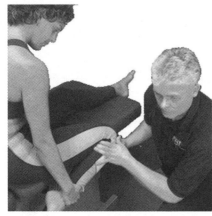

A complete or significant tearing of the ligament or meniscus usually requires corrective surgery, and cannot be treated with just soft-tissue techniques. This is particularly true of patients who want to return to a high level of activity.

Fortunately, we have found that we can effectively treat the majority of ligamentous and meniscus injuries with Active Release Techniques.

Dr. Abelson treating the lateral meniscus with ART.

Again, treatment is a matter of determining exactly which soft-tissue structures have been damaged along the kinetic chain, and then using ART to remove restrictive, adhesed tissues. All adjacent structures to the affected ligaments and meniscus must also be evaluated and treated for the presence of restrictive or binding adhesions.

Obviously, the best and easiest nonsurgical treatment is to prevent this injury from occurring at all. Often an injury to the ligaments and meniscus could have been avoided if the patient had focused on flexibility, strength, and balance exercises.

This is where ART Performance Care comes in! A large part of my practice involves the process of analyzing individuals to determine where they have soft-tissue imbalances, and then correcting these imbalances with ART. We then prescribe appropriate exercises to prevent future possible injuries.

ART and Osteoarthritis of the Knee - Osteoarthritis is often described as a disease caused by '*wear and tear*', which then leads to inflammation and all its accompanying side effects. If we can reduce that '*wear and tear*', then we can greatly decrease the rate of onset, progression, and outcome of arthritis.

Adhesions within the soft-tissues of the knee create a compressive force that reduces circulatory function, resulting in decreased blood flow, and reduced oxygen levels. This in turn causes enzymatic changes to take place that accelerate the arthritic degeneration of cartilaginous structures. In addition, the development of osteoarthritis results in a corresponding decrease in range of motion, weakened, shortened, and fibrotic musculature, and a decreased ability to absorb the shocks caused by daily walking and running.

We have found that ART is very effective at breaking the adhesions and restrictions that cause these internal pressures, and at restoring tissue movement, thereby decreasing the effects of daily gait-related '*wear and tear*'. Once these restrictions have been removed, we are then able to assign appropriate exercises that focus on restoring flexibility, strength, balance, and cardiovascular health to restore full function to the knees. ART combined with appropriate exercises can greatly reduce, and sometimes eliminate, the pain of osteoarthritis.

ART and Chondromalacia - The first thing that an ART practitioner will do when addressing the problem of Chondromalacia is a complete biomechanical evaluation to determine where the soft-tissue imbalances are located.

During this biomechanical evaluation of the patient's gait, the practitioner looks for limitations in flexion and extension of the knee and hip as well as for lateral or medial deviation of the knee. The practitioner will also look for any restrictions or lack of symmetry along the entire kinetic chain of the knee, from the feet right up to the hips.

Once the locations of these imbalances have been determined, the practitioner can apply appropriate ART procedures to release these restrictions. This is typically followed by recommendation of appropriate strengthening exercises for all the soft-tissues that surround the knee. Exercises are extremely important for resolving Chondromalacia since they help to decrease the amount of stress and pressure that is applied to the knee.

ART and Iliotibial Band Syndrome (ITBS or Runner's Knee) - All the structures in the iliotibial band's kinetic chain (above and below the area of injury), as well as the ITB itself, must perform properly in order to ensure effectiveness of the treatment. Patterns of dysfunction will continue to develop if any segment of the kinetic chain is not functioning properly.

Effective treatment of ITBS, like that of any other soft-tissue injury, requires an alteration in tissue structure to break up the restrictive cross-fiber adhesions and restore normal function to the affected soft-tissue areas. To truly resolve ITBS, every structure that crosses the lateral side of the knee must be evaluated and treated, including:

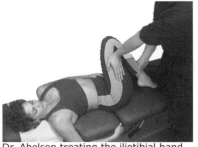

Dr. Abelson treating the iliotibial band and lateral quadricep with ART.

- The iliotibial band. Restrictive adhesions that attach the ITB to surrounding structures must be released.
- The muscles, ligaments, menisci, and knee capsule that form part of the iliotibial band's kinetic chain.
- The hip. Restrictions in the psoas, and internal and external hip rotators are the most common cause of ITBS.

Unfortunately, since most practitioners rarely evaluate and treat *all* of these structures, it is common for this condition to never fully resolve.

The actual sequence and content of each treatment can vary greatly since ITBS can be caused by dysfunctions in a variety of structures along any part of the kinetic chain. Patients may show exactly the same symptoms of ITBS, but have completely different soft-tissue injuries. This is why generic treatment methodologies often do not work when treating ITBS. The following is a list of common soft-tissue structures (other than the ITB) that may need to be addressed with an ITBS injury.

- Biceps Femoris.
- Knee Capsule.
- Collateral Ligaments.
- Gastrocnemius.
- Gluteus Medius.
- Internal and External Hip Rotators.

- Meniscus.
- Patellar Ligament.
- Peroneus Longus Muscle.
- Popliteus Muscle.
- Psoas muscle.
- Vastus Lateralis (outer hamstring).

ART and Osgood-Schlatter Disease - I do not believe that surgery is a good option for treating this condition.

I have a lot of personal experience with this condition. I had it as a child, and have a bump on my knee to prove it. My son, a budding young soccer player, is vulnerable to this condition. And in my practice, I see many active children who also show this condition, especially during soccer season.

Osgood-Schlatter Disease is not a difficult condition to treat if you know what you are doing. With ART, we complete our biomechanical analysis, and then treat all involved structures. We usually find restrictions in the:

- Quadriceps or secondary hip flexors.
- Iliacus and psoas or primary hip flexor.
- Antagonistic muscles for the quadriceps, iliacus, psoas, and hip flexors.

We usually find that the child is 80 to 90% better after just two to three ART treatments. I only wish that ART had been around when I was a kid – it would have saved me a lot of pain and grief!

A Case History

The Vancouver International Marathon has been one of my favorite races for the last 20 years. Usually a group of us train throughout the winter for this race. In our part of the world, this means running long distances at -30°F (-34°C)! So you can see that if you are willing to put up with those conditions, motivation is *not* a problem!

It was in the spring with the race date fast approaching, after one of those especially brutal winters, that a friend of mine, Tony, started to have some major knee problems. He had run numerous half-marathons before, but this was Tony's first marathon.   We had just finished our longest run prior to the race – a brutal 20 miles – when Tony had his injury.

I had been telling Tony all season that he needed to spend more time stretching his hip flexors (quadriceps and psoas). This information basically went in one ear, and out the other. Two days after our twenty mile run, and just two weeks before the Vancouver Marathon, Tony found that he could barely walk.

When I examined Tony, I found that his knee cap (patella) seemed to be tracking way over to the outside. I measured Tony's Q angle. The Q angle is way of measuring the alignment between the pelvis, leg and foot. A normal Q angle should typically fall between 18° to 22°, with men at the lower range, and women at the upper range. Tony's Q angle was way beyond normal! This gave me a pretty good indication that Tony was having some major biomechanical imbalances that were causing the problems he was having.

On further inspection, I could see that Tony's knee was not the only thing that was bothering him. (Apparently Tony had been keeping his pains to himself for several months!) I could literally follow a line of restricted tissues up from his knee to his anterior thigh, hip, low-back, mid-back, and shoulder, right up to his neck. He was a mess — but he just didn't want to admit it!

There are several common restrictions that I often see in runners, and Tony had them all.

- One part of his quadriceps (rectus femoris) was adhesed to the quadricep right underneath it (vastus intermedius). This restriction was preventing Tony from extending his leg properly.
- His iliotibial band was adhesed onto his lateral quadricep (vastus lateralis). Again, this very common restriction was causing his knee cap to move out of normal alignment, and causing all the associated muscles to torque and twist.
- The internal and external hip rotators were very tight. This is a common cause of knee problems, often leading to excessive rotation of the femur.
- The peroneus longus muscle was extremely tight. This muscle everts the foot, allows you to push off with your ankle during gait, and is involved in the support of the transverse arch of the foot.

In all, I had to release at least a dozen major restrictions before Tony could walk without considerable pain. However, after a few ART treatments, Tony was back on his feet. By race day, he was ready to go the distance, or so he told us!

This isn't the end of the story though. I ran the first fifteen miles with Tony. He did great, but then I left him since we ran at very different paces. (Running long distances at another person's pace is a good way to injure yourself.)

I thought it was a great race! I saw everyone in our running group at the finish line – with the exception of Tony. I was starting to think Tony's knee must have acted up. An hour later, and still no Tony. So I headed over to the Medical Tent, and lo and behold – there was Tony! He was hooked up to a bottle of saline, totally dehydrated, and looking like he had been dragged through a knot hole. I said, *"What happened to you?"*

Looking rather embarrassed, Tony explained that his knee was great, but it was that old geezer that knocked him out! Apparently, at about mile seventeen, Tony started to run along an older gentleman who was in his sixties. Before long, the guy was saying encouraging things to Tony like *"having trouble keeping up to the old guy, are you?"* Apparently, this completely aggravated Tony, who reacted with *"No way is this geriatric going to beat me."* Bad move, Tony!

The older gentleman had probably run over a hundred or more marathons. (I learned a long time ago to never underestimate someone just because they have a few extra years on their frame.) At mile 23, a totally exhausted Tony passed out. Luckily, as the grass stains on his forehead showed, he landed on grass. The next thing he knew, he was lying in the back of an ambulance.

On the brighter side Tony did complete his next marathon with no knee problems. He also stopped underestimating the senior citizen population!

Exercises for the Knee

Once the restrictions and adhesed tissues have been released with ART, post-treatment exercises become a critical part of the healing process, and act to ensure the repetitive strain injury does not return.

It is important to remember that these exercises are only effective if they are executed *after* the adhesions within the soft-tissue have been released by ART treatments.

Attempts to stretch muscles that are currently bound by adhesions often do not achieve the desired results. In addition, only the muscles above and below the restrictions are lengthened. The actual restricted area remains unaffected, causing further muscle imbalances and stress, resulting in the formation of yet more restrictive tissues. This is why generic stretching exercises for knee injuries seldom work.

In addition to stretching, a program of strengthening is also very important to ensure the problem does not return. The following pages depict some of the specific strengthening and stretching exercises that we recommend at our clinic for the prevention of knee injuries.

- *Partial Knee Bend - page 147.*
- *Terminal Knee Extension - page 148.*
- *Single Leg Hamstring Stretch - page 149.*
- *Stretching the Quads, Psoas, and Primary Hip Flexors - page 150.*
- *IT Band - Myofascial Release - page 151.*
- *Unilateral Partial Squat - page 152.*
- *Single Leg Lunge on a SitFitter® - page 153.*
- *Peterson Step Up - page 154.*

Partial Knee Bend - This exercise helps to develop your coordination and proprioception. It also helps you to become aware of what the proper alignment and position of the knee should be when it is bending.

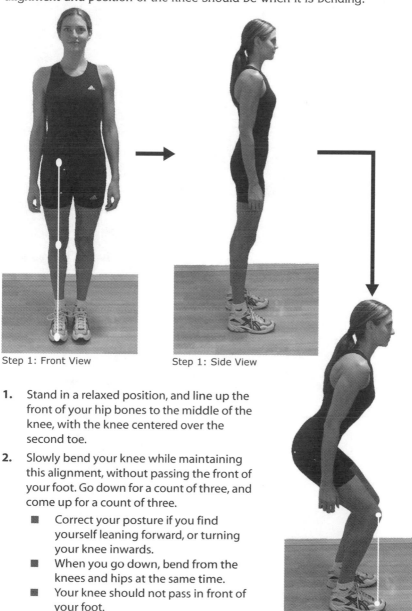

Step 1: Front View

Step 1: Side View

1. Stand in a relaxed position, and line up the front of your hip bones to the middle of the knee, with the knee centered over the second toe.

2. Slowly bend your knee while maintaining this alignment, without passing the front of your foot. Go down for a count of three, and come up for a count of three.

   ■ Correct your posture if you find yourself leaning forward, or turning your knee inwards.
   ■ When you go down, bend from the knees and hips at the same time.
   ■ Your knee should not pass in front of your foot.

3. Repeat this exercise 10 times.

4. Perform 1 to 3 sets each time.

Terminal Knee Extension - This exercise helps to stabilize the knee and strengthens the vastus medialis (one of the quadriceps). You will need a heavy medicine ball, or some other object that can be placed as a support under the knee.

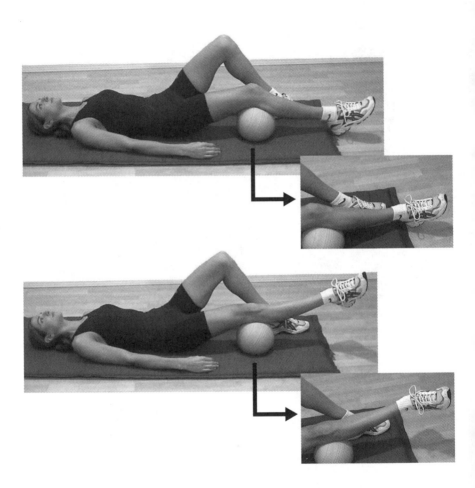

1. Lie flat on your back and place the weighted ball under your knee.
2. Rotate your foot externally.
3. Keeping the ball under your knee, slowly raise the lower part of the leg off the floor for a slow count of three, until it is straight.
4. Now lower the leg back to the floor for a slow count of three. Make sure you keep the foot rotated externally throughout this exercise.
5. Repeat this exercise 12 to 20 times for each leg.
6. Perform 1 to 3 sets each time.

Single Leg Hamstring Stretch - This exercise stretches and increases the flexibility of the gluteal fold, hamstrings, and calf muscles of the affected leg.

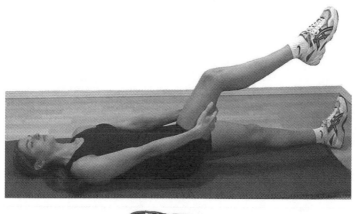

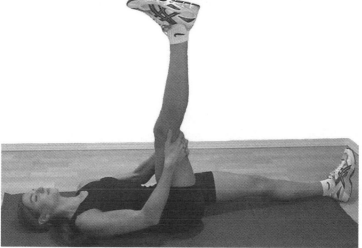

1.   Lie on your back.

2.   With both hands, reach down and clasp your leg just above the knee.

3.   Lift the leg up towards the ceiling, and pull the upper leg towards your chest, keeping the leg straight throughout the motion.

   ■   Only stretch to the point where you feel a light tension on the back of your leg. Do not overstretch.

   ■   You may feel the tension in either the upper or lower portion of the leg.

   ■   Normal range of motion is about 80 to 90 degrees.

4.   Hold the stretch for 30 seconds and repeat it for the other side.

Stretching the Quads, Psoas, and Primary Hip Flexors - This exercise lengthens and stretches the muscles in the front portion of the hip and leg.

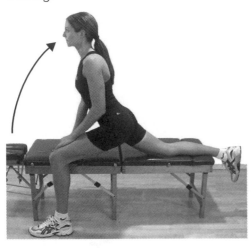

1. Lie, face down, on a table or bench. Drop the left foot flat onto the floor, keeping the right leg extended on the bench.

2. Push up with both hands to raise the upper body off the table.

3. Extend your upper body back while pushing your hip forward.

4. Maintain this position for 30 seconds to stretch the psoas of the affected leg.

5. Repeat this exercise once for each leg.

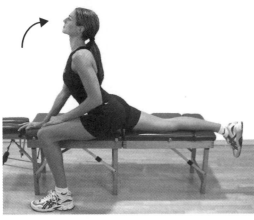

6. For an even greater stretch:
   - Start from the full stretch in step 4.
   - Bend the right leg.
   - Reach back, grasp the right foot, and pull the right foot straight towards the hip to activate and stretch the quadriceps and psoas together.

5. Repeat this exercise once for each leg.

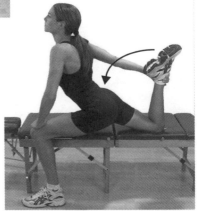

IT Band - Myofascial Release - This exercise requires the use of a foam roller. It works the iliotibial band and its supporting muscles and soft-tissues.

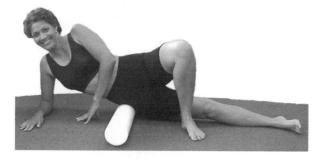

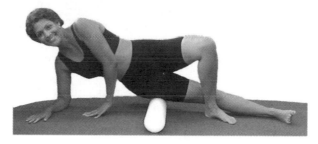

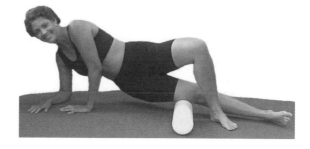

1. Lie on your side and place the foam roller under your hip, as shown in the top picture.

2. Stretch the bottom leg out straight, and bend the upper leg so that it crosses in front of the bottom leg at the knee, and the foot is flat on the floor. Brace your body off the ground with your arms.

3. Now slowly roll up and down the roller, allowing it to move from the top of your hip to the knee, and back again.

4. Repeat this exercise 15 to 20 times for both the left and right sides.

Unilateral Partial Squat - This strengthening exercise combines proprioception and balance to train the gluteal muscles to work in coordination with the muscles of the thigh. Make sure you keep your hip, knee, and second toe aligned over each other as you do this exercise.

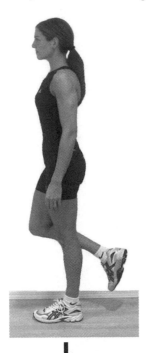

1. Stand sideways to the wall, with your shoulder about 3 to 4 inches from the wall.

   If necessary, for additional support, you can also lean lightly against the wall.

2. Bend the leg that is closest to the wall, and balance on the other leg.

3. Slowly squat down as far as you can while maintaining your alignment and balance.

   Ensure that the leg closest to the wall remains parallel to the wall throughout the exercise.

4. Come back up slowly until your leg is straight again.

5. Repeat steps 2 to 4, for 12 to 20 times for each side.

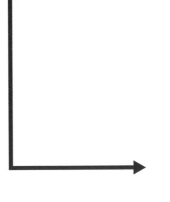

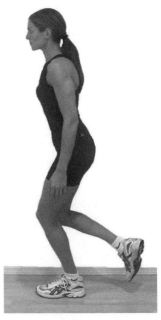

Single Leg Lunge on a SitFitter® - You will need to use a SitFitter for this exercise. This exercise stimulates and strengthens the muscles surrounding the hip, ankle, and knee. This is an advanced exercise that should only be done after you are comfortable with the Unilateral Partial Squat (see *page 152*).

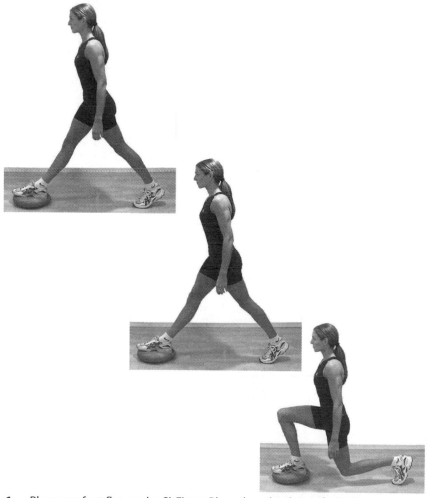

1. Place one foot flat on the SitFitter. Place the other leg as far back as you comfortably can.

2. Drop the back knee to the floor while keeping the front foot flat on the SitFitter. Ensure your posture is upright throughout the movement and that your front leg is doing all of the work.

3. Repeat this exercise 12 to 20 times for each side.

4. Perform 1 to 3 sets each time.

Peterson Step Up - You will need a thick book, such as a dictionary, for this exercise. This exercise isolates and strengthens the main stabilizers of the knee.

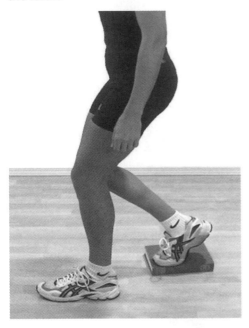

1. Position the book just behind your foot.

2. Stand with one leg straight, foot flat on the floor, and the other leg bent, with its toes resting on the book.

3. With the back foot, transfer your weight through the toe to the heel so that you raise yourself off the floor. Flatten the back foot on top of the book as you finish this movement.

   - Do not push off the front foot.
   - The front foot should be floating off the floor.
   - You will be going backward as you roll off the toe onto the heel of the back foot.

4. Slowly return to the starting position. You will be going forward as you return to starting position.

5. Repeat this exercise 12 to 20 times for each foot.

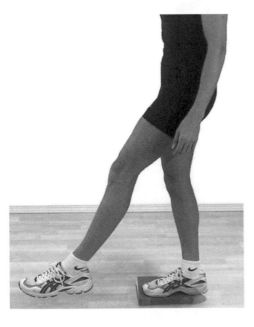

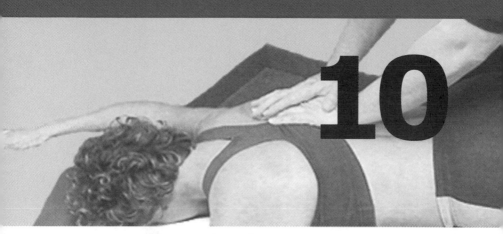

Back Pain

In this chapter

Ask yourself:

- Do you wake up at night because of back pain?
- Do you suffer from intermittent or constant pain in your back?
- Is your back pain worse in the mornings and evenings?
- Do you have pain that shoots down one or both legs?
- Can you describe your back pain as aching, tight, stiff, sore, burning, throbbing, stabbing, or pulling?
- Does your pain increase while bending, sitting, walking, or standing too long in one position?

If you answered YES to one or more of the above questions, you may have a back pain syndrome that can be helped by Active Release Techniques.

How Prevalent is Back Pain?

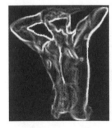 Back pain can affect anyone from children, to adults, and seniors. It is especially prevalent in individuals who lead sedentary lives. There is also an increased occurrence of back pain during the third to sixth decades of a person's life. Back pain is usually recurrent, with subsequent episodes tending to increase in severity.

Back pain is second only to the common cold as the reason for visits to the doctor. In fact, approximately 80% of the population will experience back pain at some time in their life, and 20 to 30% of the population will suffer from back pain at any given time.[1]

Back pain has put a huge burden on our health care system with annual medical costs exceeding $20 billion dollars. Back pain is the most common condition for which workers' compensation claims are filed in the United States. Studies have estimated that the cost of back pain ranges from $50 billion to $100 billion per year. It is also responsible for approximately 40% of all absences from the workplace. [2]

Caution: There are certain symptoms that could be indications for serious medical conditions which require surgery. In such cases, patients should seek immediate medical attention. Some symptoms to watch for include:

- Sudden bladder or bowel incontinence.
- Progressive weakness in the legs which could be indicative of *cauda equina syndrome*. The cauda equina is a structure formed by nerve roots below the level of spinal cord termination.
- A pulsating mass in the midline of the abdomen that is tender to touch. This could be an indication of an abdominal aortic aneurysm, a condition which must be checked for, and ruled out, before any kind of physical treatments can be applied.

1. Andersson GBJ. The epidemiology of spinal disorders. In Frymoyer JW (ed): The Adult Spine: Principles and Practice, ed 2. Lippincott-Raven, Philadelphia, 1997, pp. 93-141.
2. Guo H-R, Tanaka S, Halperin WE, et al. Am J Public Health. 1999;89:1029-1035.

About Your Back

The human back is composed of a series of complex structures that work together to allow you to perform your daily activities. When functioning correctly, your spinal musculature is incredibly strong, supportive, and flexible through all the planes of motion.

Unlike many muscles in your body, the muscles of your back are always active and in continuous use. These muscles form an essential part of your core musculature and act to:

- Help you to maintain your posture in a neutral position so that your body can effectively distribute the daily stresses placed upon it.
- Hold your torso in an upright position.
- Form the fulcrum through which the force required to move your arms and legs is generated.

A back that is not impeded in its movement, with strong flexible muscles, is essential for you to perform your normal daily tasks without adding numerous internal stresses to your body.

The Human S-Curve

The design of the human back is unique in the way it is able to distribute weight and provide balance while maintaining an upright posture.

Your back is aligned with three natural curves that form an S-shape when you are standing. The S-shaped curve of your spine oscillates during any activity (such as walking) and enables the spine to function as a shock absorber.

When your back is properly aligned, your ear, shoulder, and hip form a straight line. If the muscles of your back are weak, stressed, or constricted, you will lose this natural S shape, affect your good posture, and limit your ability to carry out normal tasks in comfort.

What makes a person more susceptible to back pain?

- Atherosclerosis
- Chronic Inflammatory Conditions
- Excess Weight
- Genetic Factors
- History of Trauma
- Infection
- Lack of Core Stability
- Medications
- Muscle Imbalances
- Normal Aging Process
- Osteoarthritis
- Osteoporosis
- Poor Musculature
- Pregnancy
- Repetitive Motion
- Scar Tissue
- Smoking

The Bones and Discs of the Back

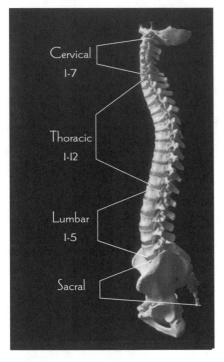

Cervical
1-7

Thoracic
1-12

Lumbar
1-5

Sacral

Your spine performs many critical functions in your back. The spine:

- Contains and protects the spinal cord.
- Allows a full range of motion. Your spine is not meant to be rigid.
- Acts as an attachment site for the muscles and ligaments of the back. Any restrictions in these attached soft-tissues can cause biomechanical imbalances that affect the functioning of the spine.

Spinal restrictions that appear within a particular range of motion, even without pain, indicate that you have some type of biomechanical dysfunction.

Discs are the spine's shock absorption mechanism and lie between, and are attached to, the vertebrae of the backbone, and form part of the front wall of the spinal canal. Discs are designed to:

- Absorb a huge amount of stress.
- Act as a hinge, permitting increased range of motion and mobility in the spine.
- Protect the spinal cord and its nerve roots.

Soft-tissue Layers of the Back

Your back is composed of multiple layers of tissue which can be divided into three major layers: superficial, intermediate, and deep. These multiple layers, combined with the musculature of the abdomen and a vast number of tendons and ligaments, form the core of your body. (See *Core Stability and Back Pain - page 165* for more information about the importance of the core in supporting the activities and actions of your back.)

When under stress, or due to repetitive actions, these core layers of soft-tissue can become *adhesed to each other*. These adhesions cause biomechanical imbalances which eventually lead to friction, inflammation, and physical dysfunctions.

In addition to the structures of the back, we must also take into account the effect that restrictions in the antagonistic or counterbalancing muscles have upon the structures of the back. The following sections describe most of the primary structures in each of the soft-tissue layers and will help you to understand some of the problems that cause back pain.

- *Superficial Structures of the Back - page 159.*
- *Intermediate Structures of the Back - page 160.*
- *Deep Structures of the Back - page 161.*
- *Counterbalancing Structures of the Spine - page 163.*

Superficial Structures of the Back

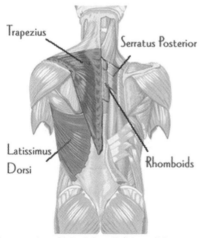

Trapezius

Serratus Posterior

Latissimus Dorsi

Rhomboids

Image courtesy of Active Release Techniques, LLC

Trapezius - The trapezius muscle raises, pulls back, and rotates the scapula. It also works to rotate the arm inward. Restrictions in this muscle lead to pains in the neck, shoulder, or mid-back.

Latissimus Dorsi - The latissimus dorsi extends the arm, pulls the arm towards the body, and rotates the arm inward. Restrictions in this muscle lead to pains in the shoulder, mid-back, or low-back.

Rhomboids Major and Minor - The rhomboids perform several major functions, including:

- Pulling the scapula back.
- Rotating the scapula.
- Stabilizing the scapula.
- Fixing the scapula position to the wall of the thoracic spine.

Typically, to relieve tension or restore normal translation to the rhomboids, the practitioner must also work on other structures both above and below the rhomboids.

Intermediate Structures of the Back

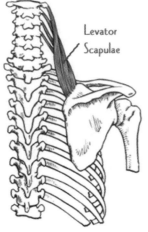

Levator Scapulae - This muscle lies just under the trapezius and acts to elevate and rotate the scapula.

Restrictions in the levator scapulae often cause tension, stiffness and pain in the neck and shoulders. Headaches are a common complaint as well.

Image courtesy of
Active Release Techniques, LLC

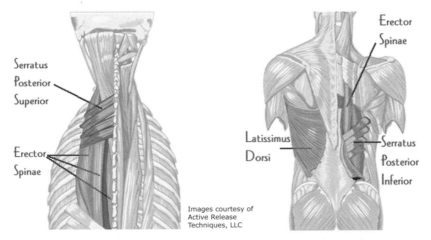

Images courtesy of
Active Release
Techniques, LLC

Serratus Posterior Superior - This muscle assists in forced inspiration. It often becomes adhesed to the rhomboids causing sharp stabbing pains in the mid-back, and restrictions in breathing.

Serratus Posterior Inferior - This muscle assists forced expiration. These muscles often become adhesed to the erector spinae resulting in restrictions in breathing, low back pain, and limited active range of motion.

Deep Structures of the Back

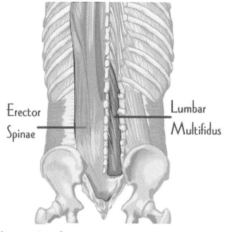

Erector Spinae

Lumbar Multifidus

Image courtesy of
Active Release Techniques, LLC

Multifidus muscles - These very deep and powerful muscles runs from the C3 vertebrae in the neck to the L5 vertebrae in the lumbar spine and act as the stabilizer for the spine, providing, through muscle contractions, approximately two-thirds of the static support in your back.

Weakness and restrictions in these muscles lead to a loss of the normal curvature of the spine and eventual muscular instability of the back.

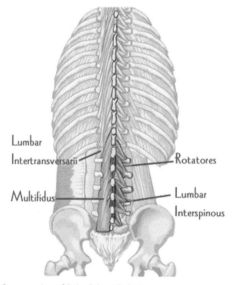

Lumbar Intertransversarii

Multifidus

Rotatores

Lumbar Interspinous

Image courtesy of Active Release Techniques, LLC

Interspinales, Intertransversarii, and Rotatores muscles - These deep structures attach directly to the spinal column and play an important role by providing:

- Support for rotational movements of the spine.
- Lateral stability for the back.
- Extension of the spinal column.

Weakness and restrictions in these muscles lead to an overall lack of core stability and chronic back pain.

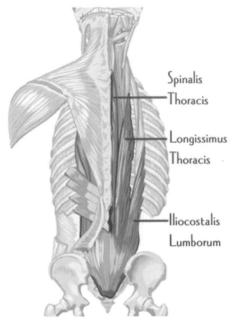

Spinalis
Thoracis

Longissimus
Thoracis

Iliocostalis
Lumborum

Image courtesy of Active Release Techniques, LLC

Erector Spinae Muscles - The muscles of the erector spinae include the:

- Spinalis muscles.
- Longissimus muscles.
- Iliocostalis muscles.

These muscles help to:

- Extend the spine.
- Laterally flex the spine.
- Link the vertebrae and enable the body to stand upright, twist, and bend.

Restrictions in these muscles result in acute and chronic back pain.

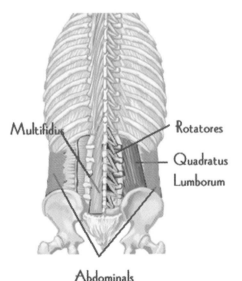

Multifidus

Rotatores

Quadratus
Lumborum

Abdominals

Image courtesy of Active Release Techniques, LLC

Quadratus Lumborum Muscle - This muscle:

- Stabilizes the floating 12th rib.
- Assists the diaphragm during the inspiration phase of breathing.
- Laterally flexes the trunk.

Restrictions in this muscle cause:

- Difficulties in breathing.
- Restrictions in lateral flexion.
- Acute and chronic low back pain.

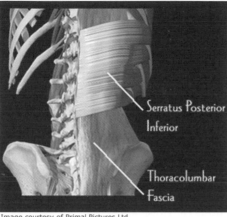

Image courtesy of Primal Pictures Ltd.
www.anatomy.tv

Serratus Posterior
Inferior

Thoracolumbar
Fascia

Thoracolumbar Fascia - This deep fascia (strong connective tissue) extends all the way from the low-back to the thoracic spine. It binds the deeper muscles of the back to the surface of the vertebrae, and surrounds the erector spinae and quadratus lumborum muscles. These two muscles then join on the side of the body to give rise to the origin of the abdominal muscles. The thoracolumbar fascia is also used to transfer forces between the legs, pelvis and spine.

Restrictions in this area result in:

■ Poor core stability.
■ Inadequate load transfer in the lower extremity leading to biomechanical imbalances.

Counterbalancing Structures of the Spine

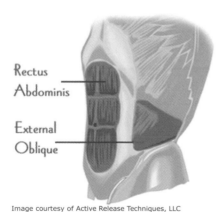

Rectus
Abdominis

External
Oblique

Image courtesy of Active Release Techniques, LLC

Internal/External Obliques & Transversus Abdominis Muscles - These muscles act as a counterbalance to the muscles of the back. They need to be strong and unrestricted in order for the back to have full range of motion, and flexibility.

These muscles transmit a compressive force, and act to increase intra-abdominal pressure that stabilizes the lumbar spine.

Restrictions in these muscles result in:

■ Lack of core stability.
■ Restricted active range of motion.
■ Acute and chronic episodes of back pain.

Ligaments

There are six primary ligaments in your back:

- Interspinous ligament.
- Ligamentum flavum.
- Supraspinatus ligament.
- Anterior longitudinal ligament.
- Posterior longitudinal ligament.
- Intertransverse ligament.

The ligaments of your back are made up of fibrous bands of connective tissue. These fibrous bands play a primary role in stabilizing your spinal cord by limiting motion as they link together bones, cartilage, and other structures. Damaged, torn, fibrotic, and shortened ligaments can result in:

- Hypermobility which can cause lack of spinal stability.
- Decreases in normal ranges of motion, which can cause imbalances that eventually lead to friction and inflammation in supporting soft-tissues.
- Overuse of supporting muscles and joints, as they attempt to compensate for ligament injury.

ART can be used to decrease the impact of ligamentous damage by releasing the fibrotic structures, and increasing circulatory function to speed healing, thus allowing the ligament to resume its function in maintaining the stability of the spine.

What Causes Back Pain

Back pain is caused by a broad range of environmental, physical, and physiological factors. Although back pain can be caused by several pathological processes, these are rare events. Back pain most commonly originates from mechanical causes such as:

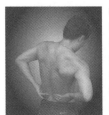

- Repetitive strain injuries.
- General lack of core stability.
- Biomechanical imbalances.
- Poor conditioning and muscle tone.
- Poor ergonomics.
- Poor posture.
- Trauma.

These primary causes are discussed in the following pages.

Repetitive Strain Injuries to the Back

What do the following factors have in common?

- Watching television.
- Sitting behind a computer for long periods of time.
- Poor workstation ergonomics.
- Weak and unconditioned muscles.
- Muscle imbalances.
- Excessive weight gain.
- Gait imbalances such as pronation or supination.
- Poor posture while sitting, standing, or performing any action.
- Jobs which require you to perform the same task over and over again.
- Driving for long periods of time.
- Standing for long periods of time.

Each one of these actions applies mechanical stress to the body which can then result in a repetitive strain injury. The basic principle of any RSI injury applies to each of the above actions:

The initial stress leads to friction,
    --> which then causes inflammation,
        --> which leads to the eventual formation of adhesions,
           --> which places stress upon the back, and
              --> results in the perpetuation of
The Cumulative Injury Cycle --- page 12.

Core Stability and Back Pain

Lack of strength, muscle imbalances, or lack of stability in the deep stabilizing muscles of the core are often associated with a variety of painful back conditions.

The foundation of your core is made up of much more than just your abdominal muscles. The core includes muscles that lie deep within your torso, and muscles that extend right up to your neck and shoulders. These muscles connect to the spine, pelvis, and shoulders to create a solid foundation of support for all the primary motions of your body.

Some of the primary core structures include:

- Multifidi muscles
- Interspinales muscles
- Intertransversarii muscles
- Rotatores muscles
- Internal/External Oblique muscles
- Transversus Abdominis muscle
- Erector Spinae muscles
- Quadratus Lumborum muscle
- Thoracolumbar fascia

When these core muscles are strong, flexible, and move freely, your body is able to compensate for, and respond to, the stresses placed upon it. When the core muscles are weak or restricted, your back becomes susceptible to a wide variety of injuries. Most commonly, due to injury or trauma, the layers of the core muscles can become adhesed together and become unable to perform their various functions.

A strong core is dependent upon an effective, restriction-free, balance between all the muscle groups that make up the core. Attempts to strengthen only some of these core muscle groups can actually increase or cause core instability and injury. These injuries may be as simple as a strain–sprain, or they may lead to more serious conditions such as herniated discs, sciatica, or long-term physical dysfunction.

ART practitioners deal with these types of problems by:

- Identifying the location and involvement of specific muscle groups through the use of a full physical examination and palpation of soft-tissues.
- Conducting a biomechanical analysis to find restrictions in motion.
- Applying specific ART protocols to remove restrictions between affected soft-tissue layers. This restores translation and movement to the layers of muscles, nerves, and ligaments. The ART protocols that are applied vary greatly with each case since every individual has specific and unique restrictions that are causing the problem.
- Applying ART protocols to structures along the back's kinetic chain to remove restrictions that may have been the original cause of the problem.

Disc Degeneration

Disc degeneration is part of the normal aging process. As we age, our discs begin to shrink due to loss of fluid within the discs. This loss of fluid in the disc leads to a decrease in the normal height of the disc, thereby decreasing the disc's ability to absorb shock.

The lack of shock absorption by the discs causes increased stress on the facet joints (a gliding joint between each vertebra) of the spine, and results in *facet joint degeneration.*

These changes may eventually cause pressure on the nerve roots (nerves that exit from the spinal cord) and may result in sciatic-type pain (pain down the leg). This condition is often referred to as *Degenerative Disc Disease.*

Disc Herniation, Protrusion, Prolapse, & Extrusion

A disc protrusion (also known as a disc bulge) occurs when the inner material of the disc starts to push out through the outer wall of the disc, creating a bulge in the disc.

In most cases this disc bulge is completely symptomless, and causes no pain or lack of function. In fact, most individuals over the age of forty have disc bulges.

Caution:	In some cases, a disc bulge or protrusion compresses a nerve and causes significant neurological dysfunction. A disc bulge that compromises the function of the nerve is normally considered to be a surgical emergency, and requires immediate surgical intervention to correct the problem. This type of condition, although rare, must be evaluated by a qualified medical practitioner.

Problems occur when these disc protrusions start to tear or fragment. A herniated disc occurs when the inner material of the disc (the nucleus pulposus) starts to push through the outer fibers of the disc (the annulus fibrosus). Most disc herniations occur at the two lower levels of the spinal column.

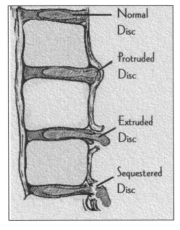

Normal Disc

Protruded Disc

Extruded Disc

Sequestered Disc

When the outer layers of a disc rupture, the inner center of the disc may move out and press upon a nerve. This condition is known as *disc prolapse* or a *protruding disc*. In such cases, the material inside the disc can sometimes extrude into the spinal canal.

In rare cases a severe prolapse will press on the nerves which control bowel and bladder function, resulting in severe muscle atrophy. These are rare events and are considered to be surgical emergencies. The majority of disc prolapses do not fit into this category.

In yet other cases, a disc may extrude right through the outer fibers of the disc, and a piece may break off completely. When this occurs, the extruded piece of disc can interfere with the function of the nearby nerves. This condition - *sequestered disc* - requires surgical intervention if it is causing neurological dysfunction, and is a problem that cannot be resolved with just soft-tissue manipulation.

However, the most important point to be made is that *most* cases that involve a disc bulge or protrusion *do not* require surgery. In fact there are a couple of common myths about disc protrusions that we should consider:

■ **The first myth** is that the presence of a large disc protrusion – as often seen on MRI or CAT scan images – is an indication that this problem cannot be resolved with conservative care (non-surgical).

In reality, research is showing the exact opposite to be true. The larger the disc protrusion, the greater the reduction in protrusion size after conservative treatment. [1]

■ **The second myth** is that the extruded and sequestered disc fragments are less likely to resolve than the contained protrusions.

[1.] Dullerud R, Nakstad PH. CT CHANGES AFTER CONSERVATIVE TREATMENT FOR LUMBAR DISC HERNIATION. Acta Radiologica, 1994;35:415-419.

In actuality, the migrating fragments actually resolve more frequently and faster than the contained protrusions.[1] [2]The reason for this is, the larger the disc protrusion, the greater the degree of inflammation around the protrusion. Once disc fragments have broken off, inflammation around the fragments and the disc decreases, allowing the body to reabsorb the fragments more easily.[3]

Note: MRIs are commonly used as a diagnostic tool for identifying where a disc protrusion is occurring. However, a protruding disc is not always the true cause of the pain and discomfort. To arrive at a proper diagnosis, it is very important that the practitioner correlate the MRI results against the comprehensive physical examination and clinical symptoms exhibited by the patient.

Resolving Disc Protrusions and Herniations - Anything that can be done to remove biomechanical stress from the back can benefit the patient. During the acute stage of the injury anti-inflammatories and ice are useful, but only at a symptomatic level. They do not resolve the actual dysfunction – the inflammation, adhesive restrictions, and tissue hypoxia that result from the stresses caused by disc protrusion and herniation.

Since each of these restrictions exerts a constant, ongoing stress upon the structures of the back, the key to addressing many of these disc-related conditions is the application of ART to release all restrictions along the back's kinetic chain. Once the restrictions between these soft-tissue structures have been released, it is important to restore strength, flexibility, and balance to both the primary structures involved, and their antagonists (opposing structures). In addition to ART, I generally recommend the application of spinal manipulation techniques to normalize spinal mechanics. By normalize, I refer to the restoration of normal ranges-of-motion to the spinal joints through all planes of motion.

We have successfully treated and resolved hundreds of disc cases by using ART. Only the rare and extreme cases require surgery to resolve disc-related problems.

[1.] Komori H, Shinomiya K, Nakai O, Yamaura I, Takeda S, Furuya K. THE NATURAL HISTORY OF HERNIATED NUCLEUS PULPOSUS WITH RADICULOPATHY. Spine, 1996;21:225-229.
[2.] Ikeda T, Nakamura T Kikuchi T, Senda H, Tagagi K. Pathomechanism Of Spontaneous Regression Of The Herniated Lumbar Disc: Histologic And Immunohistochemical Study. J Spinal Disord, 1996;9:136-140.
[3.] Maigne J-Y, Deligne L. Computed Tomographic Follow-up Study Of 21 Cases Of Nonoperatively Treated Cervical Intervertebral Soft Disc Herniation. Spine, 1994;19:189-191.

Sciatica

Sciatica is a common form of back pain. The classical definition of Sciatica refers to pain along the large sciatic nerve – which runs from the lower back and down the back of each leg.

The pain can vary in location; it may go down your buttocks, through your thigh, down the back of your leg, or right down to the foot and heel.

The majority of the medical community believes that Sciatica is a result of pressure upon the sciatic nerve caused by a herniated disc in the spine. Through Active Release Techniques, however, it has been revealed that Sciatica is more often caused by *peripheral* nerve entrapments. The most common sciatic nerve entrapment sites include adhesion of the sciatic nerve:

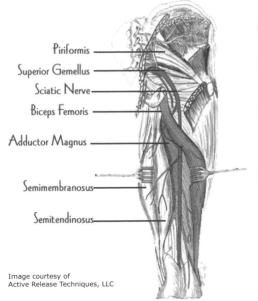

Piriformis

Superior Gemellus

Sciatic Nerve

Biceps Femoris

Adductor Magnus

Semimembranosus

Semitendinosus

Image courtesy of
Active Release Techniques, LLC

- Between the muscles of the hamstrings.
- Between the adductor magnus and hamstring muscles.
- At the superior gemellus muscle where the sciatic nerve passes over the muscle.
- At the piriformis muscle where the sciatic nerve passes under or through the muscle.

The key to resolving Sciatica is in the release of restrictions at all possible nerve entrapment sites, along the entire length of the sciatic nerve. Complete resolution of Sciatica cannot be achieved if the nerve remains trapped at any location along its length. This is where Active Release Techniques excels: it can be used to *find* each of these entrapment sites, and then, to *release* their restrictions.

Facet Joint Syndrome

Facet joint pain is generally chronic or ongoing in nature. Often the back pain caused by facet joints is only felt on one side of the spine. The pain, described as deep, sharp, and aching, usually occurs about one- to one-and-a-half inches on either side of the spine. Sometimes the pain travels down to the gluteus muscles or thigh area.

This condition is made worse by bending towards the affected side, or by extending the spine (backward bending). Problems are exacerbated by long periods of sitting or standing.

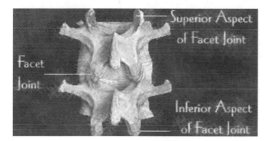

The facet joints are located between each vertebra. These joints help to guide the movement and articulation of the spine, to limit extreme movements, and to provide spinal stability.

The facet joints are each enclosed within a joint capsule that allows them to glide smoothly as the spine moves through its various ranges of motion.

Facet joint pain is usually due to long-term changes within the joint as a response to increased stress, poor core stability, or as a response to a series of seemingly minor traumas to the joint. These changes result in:

- Inflammation of the facet joints.
- Degeneration of the facet joint due to disc degeneration and the resulting lack of shock absorption by the disc.
- Increase in joint size due to remodeling of the bone.

The key to resolving Facet Joint Syndrome is to release all restricted structures, restore flexibility and strength, and ensure that the muscles of the back are symmetrical and balanced through all planes of motion. In addition, Facet Joint Syndrome often involves entrapment of nerves within adjacent soft-tissue structures.

The exact structures that are treated with ART will vary from patient to patient, since the same symptoms can occur even when different structures are involved.

Traditional Treatments for Back Pain

Traditional treatments for back pain vary greatly depending upon the practitioner, location of the practice, his or her training, and the level of diagnostic research that is carried out. This book is not intended to provide a detailed discussion about all the available treatment methods, but will instead touch upon a few aspects that we believe are either common or important concepts. These include:

- The Importance of Physical Examinations --- page 172.
- The value of X-rays for pain diagnosis --- page 174.
- The value of MRI --- page 175.
- About the effectiveness of bed rest --- page 176.
- The effectiveness of pain medications --- page 176.
- Is surgery really required? --- page 177.

The Importance of Physical Examinations

As we just discussed, the majority of back pain is caused by some type of mechanical problem. A thorough physical examination can help to rule out any pathological causes, and can help the practitioner identify the true physical/mechanical causes of the problem.

Unfortunately, I find that most doctors do **not** perform very complete physical examinations, either because they are too busy or because they don't fully understand the mechanics of back injuries. An inadequate physical examination often leads to advice like:

> 'Take these pills for a couple of days and give me a call if the pain gets worse.'

This is *extremely limited* advice – which rarely resolves the true cause of the back pain – leading to possible drug-related side-effects that often result in further physiological and biomechanical problems.

A good and complete physical examination should include:

- A check of your vitals including blood pressure, heart rate, and breathing.

- A neurological evaluation that tests your deep tendon reflexes, evaluates your sensory responses, and checks muscle strength.

- An orthopedic evaluation. These orthopedic tests can point the practitioner towards the affected soft-tissue structures. It should be noted that these tests provide only a limited amount of information. Complete reliance on *just* these tests can lead to invalid conclusions.

- A thorough *hands-on* evaluation with palpation to determine exactly which structures are involved in causing the back pain. The practitioner needs to be able to *feel* which structures have lost their ability to translate over or through one another. This includes the identification of which nerves are entrapped, where they are entrapped, and which tissues are restricting them.

- An evaluation of the back's range of motion.

- Motion or biomechanical analysis. After the hands-on palpation, this is by far the most important part of the physical examination, and quickly provides a great deal of information to the practitioner about exactly which soft-tissue structures are restricted.

  The biomechanical analysis may include having the patient walk, sit, and stand while the doctor observes relative motion, gait, and posture. Obviously the practitioner must be trained in biomechanics to perform this aspect of the physical examination.

The value of X-rays for pain diagnosis

I think that often, many practitioners are too quick in ordering X-rays for patients with back pain. I rarely need to order X-rays for patients with soft-tissue injuries, except:

- When the patient has suffered from some type of trauma.
- When the patient has been in a motor vehicle accident.
- When I need to rule out some type of pathological process such as fracture, infection, severe degeneration, or osteoporosis.

X-rays are important for identifying problems with the bones of the body, but are rarely useful for identifying the types of soft-tissue problems that normally cause back pain. In fact, it is quite common that X-rays show variations of so-called degeneration (normal wear) in individuals who are completely pain-free.

We have found that X-rays do not provide any positive diagnostic information for at least 90% of our back patients.

Discs, nerves, muscles, tendons, ligaments, and fascia are all soft-tissues that do not show up on X-rays. These soft-tissues are the cause of the majority of cases of back pain, but injuries and restrictions in these structures do not show up on X-rays.

Since these injuries do not appear on X-rays, patients are often told that the problem is "*all in their head.*" This statement is plainly ridiculous since most back pain is caused by soft-tissue injuries, not by problems with the bones.

X-rays are only useful as diagnostic tools when trying to rule out pathological processes, trauma, or injury from motor vehicle accidents.

What about Bone Spurs?

Practitioners frequently point to bone spurs that show up in X-rays, and claim a correlation between those bone spurs and the pain that the patient is feeling.

Bone spurs do *not* normally cause back pain. Rather, they are an indication of degenerative arthritis. As our spinal joints degenerate during the normal aging process, the body tries to decrease the resulting pressure by expanding the surface area of the spinal joints by forming bone spurs.

The only time bone spurs cause a physical problem is when they compress upon a nerve.

Interestingly, many bone spurs have been shown to dissolve once the soft-tissue restrictions causing the back pain have been removed.

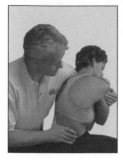

The bottom line is that most routine X-rays of the spine provide little diagnostic value. The spinal abnormalities detected with X-rays often have nothing to do with the symptoms that the patient is experiencing.

In fact, it is the information I obtain during the patient's physical examination that generally determines my treatment program.

The value of MRI

MRI (Magnetic Resonance Imaging) uses radio waves and a strong magnetic field to provide clear and detailed pictures of internal organs and tissues. The MRI shows nerves, muscles, tendons, ligaments, and discs, as well as the bones of the body.

Under the right circumstances, MRI is a good diagnostic tool which can provide detailed information about the condition of the soft-tissues. However, in most cases, MRIs are neither needed nor justified.

MRIs are often ordered due to practitioner fears of malpractice or to justify unnecessary surgery. Again, as with X-rays, an abnormal finding on an MRI may be nothing more than an indication of the normal degenerative changes that occur due to aging. Many of these so-called abnormalities are commonly found in people who have absolutely no back pain.

An MRI will give you a better picture, not necessarily a better diagnosis. For example, an MRI may show where a disc is protruding, but will not show the cause of the disc protrusion.

All MRI findings must be correlated with the symptom patterns and with the results of the physical examination. It is only when these readings correlate that the practitioner can be assured that his or her diagnosis correctly reflects the true problem.

About the effectiveness of bed rest

It amazes me that there are still numerous doctors who tell their patients to '*stay in bed*' for extended periods of time as a means to treat low back pain. Except for extreme cases, bed rest is one of the worst things you could do!

Extended bed rest causes muscle atrophy, a decrease in circulation, and an increase in inflammation due to histamine pooling. It is very important to continue your daily living activities. The sooner you return to activity and exercise, the sooner you will get better. As the saying goes - *What you don't use, you lose!*

The effectiveness of pain medications

Practitioners frequently prescribe pain-numbing medications, anti-inflammatories, or cortisone shots to combat back pain.

I am not against taking certain medications in order to deal with an acute episode of back pain. Certain medications can be very useful in controlling the symptoms during the initial stages of acute back pain. These medications can also help to reduce inflammation and stop muscle spasticity.

Although these drugs are useful in hiding the symptoms of the problem (the pain), they do not address or resolve the underlying cause of the problem - the soft-tissue injuries that caused the original problem.

Unfortunately, when taken for extended periods of time, these drugs also come with numerous side effects (kidney, liver, and gastrointestinal problems). In cases of chronic pain, these drugs can also lead to dependency and addiction. Long-term use of muscle relaxants can lead to depression.

The best solution continues to be the removal of the actual cause of the back pain, which in most cases, includes restrictions and adhesions in the soft-tissue structures.

Is surgery really required?

Sometimes surgery is necessary. In fact, I myself have undergone a microdiscectomy – a procedure that removes a fraction of a disc that is impinging upon a nerve – when I found myself suffering from progressive neurological deficits that left me in excruciating pain.

However, I do believe that surgery should always be the last option to be considered, except when a condition exists that can cause severe damage. This includes:

- Spinal tumors.
- Urinary or bowel incontinence.
- Progressive neurological deficits.

Such conditions are very rare, can only be addressed through surgery, and should be considered to be surgical emergencies that require immediate care.

Often, even when an MRI shows damage to a disc, 85-90% of these patients can recover fully without surgery. Interestingly, MRIs have also shown that over a period of time, the herniated parts of the disc often shrink and are reabsorbed by the body. This negates the most common cause, or justification, for surgery. [1]

Different surgical procedures have varying risk rates. If you are considering surgery, take the time and effort to obtain a second opinion. If your doctor seems to be threatened by the idea of a second opinion, then get a new doctor!

Don't let anyone scare you into surgery. Generally, for most cases, you will have the time you need to try alternatives to surgery. Until you try the more conservative treatments, you cannot know that *'your back pain will never go away without surgery'*.

Try the alternatives...you may be pleasantly surprised at the results!

---

[1] Workplace Health and Safety, September 2002, Government of Alberta, Human Resources and Employment

When do doctors recommend surgery?

Sadly, the reasons for performing back surgery can have little to do with the actual need for surgery. The frequency with which back surgeries are recommended can vary greatly depending upon:

Where you live – As sad as this sounds, the rates of surgery, for the same conditions, varies by more than **800%** depending on where in the country you live. [1]

Your doctor's training – The doctor's level of training and place of education greatly affects the likelihood of whether or not he will recommend surgery.

Insurance coverage – Funny how this works, but when a surgical procedure is not covered, then it is usually *not recommended*.

1. Medical versus Surgical Treatment for Low Back Pain: Evidence and Clinical Practice, Effective Clinical Practice, September/October 1999. 2:218-227

How ART Resolves Back Injuries

ART practitioners start by obtaining a comprehensive history, performing a full physical examination, and conducting a biomechanical analysis of the patient's gait, posture, and normal actions. This biomechanical analysis is used to determine exactly where restrictions are located in the back.

Once these primary restrictions have been identified, the practitioner then checks the back's kinetic chain (legs, arms, and neck) to find restrictions in the areas that may affect the back. Typically, the ART practitioner will first evaluate your 'core' since this is where the majority of back problems originate.

ART Can Resolve Back Pain

ART has been used to successfully treat the following types of back pain and back injuries:

- Soft-tissue injuries.
- Disc problems.
- Sciatica.
- Facet joint syndrome.
- Fibromyalgia.
- Back pain due to pregnancy.
- Sacroiliac dysfunctions.
- Scoliosis.
- Back pain due to sports injuries.

After the biomechanical evaluation, the practitioner applies the appropriate ART protocols to release these restrictions and restore or improve function. During these procedures, the practitioner:

- Uses a highly developed sense of touch to palpate and find the soft-tissue restrictions.
- Identifies the direction in which the restrictive adhesions have been laid down.
- Physically *works* the tissue back to its normal texture, tension, and length by using various hand positions and soft-tissue manipulation methods.

Using this process, the practitioner is able to release soft-tissue restrictions along the entire length of the structure. Entrapped nerves are released so that they can now translate and move freely through the muscles, fascia, and other soft-tissue structures that were entrapping them.

When executed properly, the ART process treats and resolves the root cause of the injury (unlike other methods which simply hide the symptoms).

By using ART to restore the relative translation and movement across each other of the multiple layers of soft-tissue in the back, we commonly see complete resolution of a back problem within just six to eight treatments.

Once these restrictions have been resolved, we are able to prescribe specific exercises which help our patients strengthen, stretch, and restore muscle tone in the affected soft-tissues.

My Own Story

When it comes to treating back pain, I have some very strong opinions about what works, and what doesn't! My opinions are based on more than clinical experience. My personal experience with back pain began when I began to compete as a triathlete, and concluded with a disc herniation in my lower back that was accompanied by a very severe case of sciatica.

Years ago, I ran a very different type of practice than I do today. As a Chiropractor, I adjusted hundreds of patients every week, placed them on exercise programs, and achieved what I thought were good results. Now, when I look back at those results, I realize that I had no idea what *good results* really meant.

Like most Chiropractors, I treated back pain with a variety of standard manipulation techniques. In most cases, our patients (after an extended period of care) got to a point where they experienced little or no pain – as long as they received regular maintenance care (once or twice per month).

At that time, I didn't understand that the need for ongoing maintenance care is an indication that the root cause of the problem has not been resolved.

However, there is nothing like personal experience to change your perspective. I have always been a very physically active person, and for the last twenty years, marathons, triathlons, and rock climbing have been a large part of my active life.

So it wasn't the easiest thing to take when I woke up one day and found that I could not even take ten steps without collapsing on the floor from excruciating back pain.

I demonstrated all the classic neurological signs of a prolapsed or extruded disc, including the severe sciatic pain that felt like a continuous burning knife stabbing from my low back to the bottom of my foot. Nothing I tried could relieve this pain, not Chiropractic adjustments, not massage therapy, not stretching, not ice packs, not even medications. To make things worse, I was starting to manifest some of the progressive neurologic deficits which indicated a need for immediate surgery.

And surgery is exactly what I needed. I received a partial microdiscectomy at the L5/S1 vertebra. Eventually, several weeks after the operation, I was able to return to my practice.

However, I continued to experience some discomfort and pain, and a considerable decrease in strength, and I found that my left leg and foot were still numb and lacking sensation. The neurosurgeon told me that some of these feelings would return within a period of six months to a year, and that the numbness would fade. However, I could not expect to regain full strength in that leg.

Unwilling to accept this diagnosis, I started on an aggressive program of exercise, massage therapy, and physical manipulation. After several months, it became obvious to me that neither the surgery, nor the other treatments, were resolving my problem. This was a very frustrating feeling for someone who has always been so active.

About one year after my operation, I started to learn and practice Active Release Techniques (ART). During this time the weakness, numbness, and lack of function in my back and legs continued to bother me, and continued to affect my function.

Fortunately, during one of my ART training courses, I asked Dr. Michael Leahy (the developer of ART) to take a look at my back. To tell the truth, I didn't really expect too much to change.

Dr. Leahy performed a short gait analysis, and examined my back and legs. He indicated there were several adhesions in my hip muscles and hamstrings which were impinging on my sciatic nerve.

When he started to apply ART protocols to these affected areas, I felt as if I had just blown my disc again. I felt the original pain pattern shooting down my leg, severe leg cramping, and the stabbing knife-like pain. I found myself wondering, *"What the hell is he doing to me."* The last thing I wanted was to be back in a hospital.

However, when I got up from the table, I was surprised to see how much looser and stronger my leg felt. Two subsequent ART treatments found me completely without low back or sciatic pain. Additionally, the ongoing numbness in my leg was gone, and much of my strength had returned.

Being both the eternal skeptic and optimist, I decided to go for a run, something I had been unable to do since my surgery. I could not believe how strong I was. For several years prior to surgery, I had found that my running speed had decreased considerably. I had assumed that the change was just part of aging! But I was wrong! Not only could I run again, but I ran better than I had for years.

Neither the pain nor the numbness has returned over the last few years. Not even the stresses of marathon or full-length Ironman Triathlon training has caused any regression.

This experience led me to ask some important questions:

- What was the real cause of my sciatic pain?
- Was the prolapsed disc the primary cause of the problem, or was the prolapsed disc a secondary result of peripheral nerve entrapment?
- And most importantly, just how effectively was I treating patients with similar sciatic/disc pain, or those with other forms of back pain?

Learning From My Experience

My own experience with back pain has shown me that back pain of a mechanical origin is often caused by entrapment and restriction of soft-tissues (nerves, muscles, ligaments, and so on). I have also become convinced that any effective therapy must first address the release of these entrapped tissues in order to successfully treat the underlying cause of this condition.

In my own case, the severe sciatica was actually caused by structures further down the kinetic chain, including:

- Soft-tissue entrapments within the external rotators of my hip and within my hamstrings.
- Sciatic nerve entrapments in multiple locations including between the hamstrings, between the adductor and hamstring muscles, and between the superior gemellus and piriformis muscles.

The disc problem, for which I required surgery, was actually only a secondary problem.

I am not so blind or single-minded as to think that my own case will apply to everyone. However, since then, I have successfully treated hundreds of patients suffering from various forms of back pain, and obtained similar and successful results.

Now, when I perform ART for a back injury, I consider the relative translation of all the soft-tissues involved. Not just in the area of pain, but within the entire kinetic chain of the affected area.

A Case History - Back Pain

During 2001, I had the pleasure of working with the ART Ironman Team at both the Penticton Canadian Ironman Championships and at the Kona, Hawaii Ironman World Championships. The ART Ironman Teams consisted of ART practitioners from the fields of Chiropractic, Physiotherapy, Medicine, Massage, and Sports Training.

Many remarkable athletes attended our outdoor clinics at these triathlon events to receive ART treatments. We witnessed many amazing and inspiring recoveries.

One case stands out in my mind. Sandy was a 27-year-old woman from California, who had trained for six years to be at the Penticton Ironman. Two weeks prior to the Ironman she began to experience severe low back and hip pain on her right side. She had seen her MD and Chiropractor prior to coming to the triathlon, without any improvement. In fact, her condition had been getting worse.

She came to see us at the Penticton ART Ironman Clinic just two days before the Ironman event. She was in extreme pain, limping, and barely able to walk. Despite her pain, she was determined to at least start the race and do her best at completing the event. Sandy had a history of ankle sprains, shin splints, knee trouble, and occasional back pain. She underwent maintenance Chiropractic care for these conditions, which never resolved the problems, but did keep them under control between visits. Due to ongoing pain during her training, she had received regular Chiropractic treatments for over six years.

I conducted a biomechanical gait analysis and found several areas of restriction in her body, and was also able to identify numerous soft-tissue structures that needed to be treated. It should be noted that Sandy found it very painful to walk even the short 50 yards required for the gait analysis.

- We started with the tibialis anterior and peroneus longus muscles which are often involved in ankle sprains. Both of these muscles act as stabilizers for the ankle and are often injured during inversion sprains.

- The posterior area of the knee (over the popliteus muscle behind the knee) was extremely tender to palpation. This muscle works hard to provide rotational stability to the knee. After releasing the restrictions in this muscle, I found that her right knee was now correctly aligned with her foot.

- We then worked the iliotibial band, gluteus medius, and gluteus minimus. Restrictions in these structures are often the cause of hip pain and low back pain.

- Finally we focused our treatments upon the primary hip flexors – the psoas and iliacus muscles. These critical core muscles in the abdomen are a key cause of back and hip pain, but are rarely treated. Sandy noted a drastic reduction in pain almost immediately after our work on her psoas and iliacus.

Our Results . . .

We then repeated our gait analysis by having Sandy run down to the end of the field and back. She was able to do this run with just minor discomfort. The difference was incredible – in fact – it was difficult to believe we were looking at the same patient. There was no deviation of the lower extremity, she had straight knees, fluid motion through the hips and SI joints (hip joints), and a noticeable reduction in her hyperlordotic curve (low back spinal curvature).

Sandy returned the next day with a very big smile. She had *no pain* for the first time in six years. We repeated the ART procedures and saw even more improvement.

During the Ironman Triathlon, I had the great pleasure of watching Sandy cross the finish line after her 140.6 mile ordeal. And most profoundly rewarding, after crossing the line in a state of exhaustion, Sandy took the time to walk up to me to thank me for helping her get there!

Exercises for the Back

Once the restrictions and adhesed tissues have been released with ART, post-treatment exercises become a critical part of the healing process, and act to ensure the RSI does not return.

It is important to remember that exercises are only effective if they are executed *after* the adhesions within the soft-tissue have been released by ART treatments.

Attempts to stretch muscles that are currently bound by adhesions often do not achieve the desired results. In addition, only the muscles above and below the restrictions are lengthened. The actual restricted area remains unaffected, causing further muscle imbalances and stresses, and resulting in the formation of yet more restrictive tissues. This is why generic stretching exercises for back pain seldom work.

In addition to stretching, a program of strengthening is also very important to ensure the problem does not return. The following pages depict some of the specific strengthening and stretching exercises that we recommend at our clinic for the prevention of back pain.

Tummy Tuck - This is an important exercise for individuals suffering from back pain. This exercise develops your sense of muscle awareness and works the transversus abdominus, multifidus, and the entire pelvic floor. These muscles act as your body's weight belt, supporting and strengthening all actions.

Typically these deep muscles are deactivated or affected in individuals suffering from back pain. By reactivating these muscles, you restart the force-coupling relationships between these muscles. This exercise helps you to first isolate and find these deep muscles, and then shows you how to activate these deep abdominal muscles.

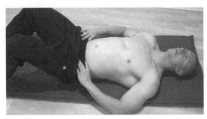 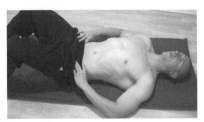

1.   Lie on your back and relax your stomach muscles.

2.   Isolate and find the transversus muscle by:
     ■   Finding and placing your forefinger upon the hip bone.
     ■   Moving your hand towards the center of your body by one inch.
     ■   Moving downwards by another inch to locate the muscle. The muscle should feel flaccid and relaxed when you touch it at this time.

3.   Create a concave stomach by pulling your navel down towards your spine. Keep your spine neutral and do *not* press the low back into the floor.
     ■   This action activates the deepest abdominal muscles.
     ■   This is a subtle movement, and may take some time to achieve.
     ■   You are looking for a maximum of 25% to 30% voluntary contraction.
     ■   It is important to keep the contraction light; do not push too hard since too much force can actually cause a dysfunction in these muscles.

4.   Hold the contraction for 10 seconds while breathing through the diaphragm.

5.   Relax, and repeat the exercise 5 to 10 times.

The Cobra - This exercise elongates the anterior joints surrounding the muscles of the spine and promotes correct spinal movement for stiff or dysfunctional low backs.

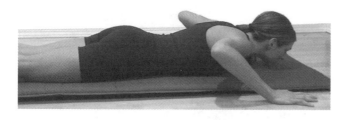

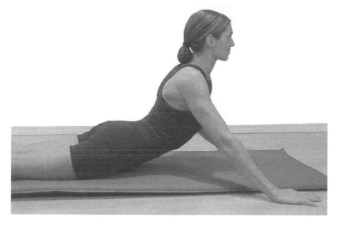

1. Lie on your stomach, palms flat on the ground, in line with your shoulders, in a push-up position.

2. Use your arms to push your upper body off the ground.
   - ■ Exhale as you push the upper body off the ground. This allows the abdominals to relax.
   - ■ Ensure that your hips, pelvis, and legs stay on the ground throughout this movement.

3. Allow the abdominals to relax as you inhale and return to the ground.

4. Repeat the exercise 10 times in a continuous smooth motion with no pauses between the actions.

Stretching the Erector Spinae - This excellent stretch helps to relax and open up the muscles of the posterior chain. You will need an exercise ball for this exercise.

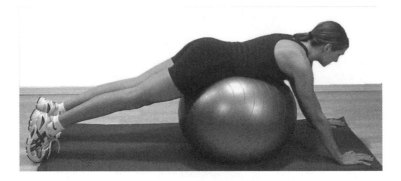

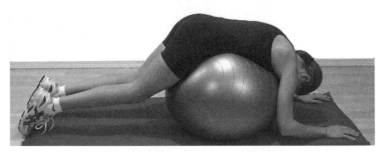

1. Lie on your stomach on a ball, with your arms and legs extended over the ball, and touching the ground.

2. Allow your body to relax over the ball – exhaling as you do this movement.

3. Remain relaxed over the ball for 30 seconds, or until tension is released in the affected area.

4-Point Kneeling - This exercise helps you to develop your sense of balance and proprioception, as well as to activate and strengthen your deep abdominal muscles.

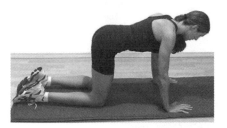

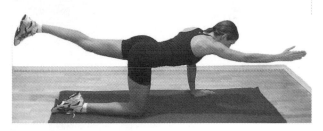

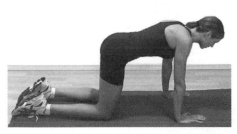

1. Kneel on all fours on the floor, with a neutral spine, and with your back parallel to the floor.

    Ensure your weight is distributed evenly across all four limbs.

2. Set your deep abdominal muscles – by drawing your navel up towards the spine. See Tummy Tuck --- page 186 for details.

    You must maintain this abdominal setting throughout the exercise.

3. Extend one arm and the opposite leg out and hold for 10 seconds.
    - Do not allow your back to rotate.
    - Do not allow your weight to shift.
    - Maintain a neutral spine, without any additional curvature, while doing this movement.

4. Return to starting position, and reset your deep abdominal muscles.

5. Repeat this exercise for the other side.

6. Carry out four to six sets (right and left sides) of this exercise, maintaining neutral spine, and setting the deep abdominals each time.

Strengthening the Core and Stabilizing the Posterior Chain - This exercise stabilizes the pelvis and strengthens the posterior chain of muscles in the back (gluteals, hamstrings, erector spinae, multifidus, and deep abdominal muscles). This exercise also trains the multifidus in the pelvis to avoid unnecessary rotations during loading.

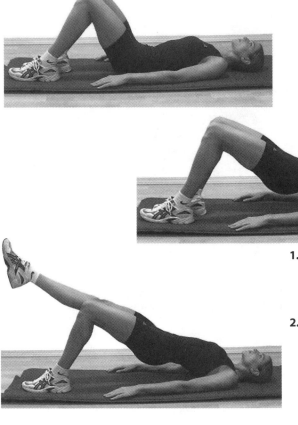

1. Lay on your back with your knees bent and your arms by your side.

2. Set your deep abdominal muscles by drawing your *navel* down towards your spine. See Tummy Tuck --- page 186 for details.

3. Slowly lift your hips up for a count of 3 seconds.

4. Lift and extend one leg up – taking 3 seconds to lift.
   Do *not* allow the pelvis to rotate as you perform this movement as this will negate the positive effects of this exercise.

5. Hold the leg up for 3 seconds, then lower the leg – taking 3 seconds to lower the leg.

6. Lower your body to the ground for a count of 3 seconds.

7. Repeat 8 to 10 times for each leg, ensuring that you maintain a neutral spine, and activation of the deep abdominal muscles with each repetition.

Bridging - This is a strengthening exercise for the muscles of your back and abdominals, specifically those that are designed to act as stabilizers of the spine.

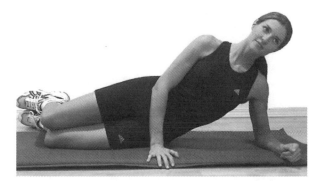

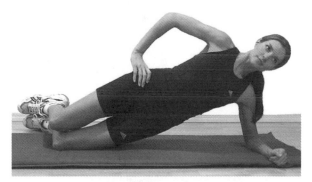

1. Lie on your side with your knees bent and your body raised off the ground, supported by your elbow and knees.

2. Set your deep abdominal muscles by drawing your navel down towards your spine. See Tummy Tuck --- page 186 for details.
    - Ensure your spine remains in a neutral position.

3. Raise your hips off the ground.
    - Keep your navel tucked in.
    - Align head, torso, hips, and legs into a straight line.
    - Your body should remain straight, with no curves sideways, forwards, or backwards.

4. Hold this pose for 10 to 60 seconds – depending upon your endurance and ability.

5. Repeat the exercise for the other side for the same amount of time.

Dead Bug - This exercise is used to promote strength, endurance, and ability of the deep abdominal muscles. Moving your limbs enables these muscles to work in coordination with the muscles in other parts of your body.

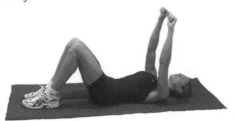
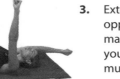

1. Lay on your back, arms reaching for the ceiling, and legs bent at the hips, as shown in the first image.

2. Set your deep abdominal muscles by drawing your navel down towards your spine. See Tummy Tuck --- page 186 for details.

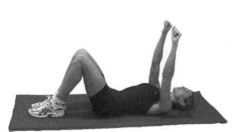
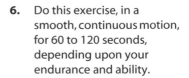

3. Extend your arm and opposite leg while maintaining the setting of your deep abdominal muscles.

4. Return to dead bug pose.

5. Repeat this exercise for the other side.

6. Do this exercise, in a smooth, continuous motion, for 60 to 120 seconds, depending upon your endurance and ability.

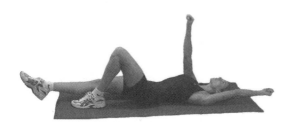

FAQ - Frequently Asked Questions

In this chapter

Benefits of ART!

- Who can benefit from ART? ---- page 194.
- How can ART improve athletic performance? ---- page 195.
- I have had an acute injury; how long must I wait before I can begin ART treatments? ---- page 196.
- Is there a difference between ART and other myofascial techniques? ---- page 196.
- What if my doctor recommends surgery? ---- page 197.

Who can benefit from ART?

Anyone who suffers from any type of repetitive strain injury – from the athlete, to the office worker, to the home-keeper – can be helped by treatments with Active Release Techniques. In addition, ART is an effective tool for improving athletic and sport performance.

Many professional athletes have come to regard ART very highly for its almost miraculous results in the treatment of serious injuries. For example, hockey player Gary Roberts was initially unable to return to hockey after two neck surgeries failed to correct his dizzy spells. He credits Dr. Leahy and ART with correcting the problem, and for allowing him to return to playing hockey.

ART should be your first choice if you have any type of repetitive strain injury since it is able to resolve the majority of these cases without the use of invasive techniques like surgery, and can do so with almost no side effects (aside from a temporary tenderness of the soft-tissues).

Review the following sections of this book for a better understanding of RSIs and how ART can help resolve these problems:

- Why is RSI a Problem? ---- page 1.
- The Specifics of RSI ---- page 7.
- About Active Release Techniques (ART) ---- page 15.

How can ART improve athletic performance?

Performance of any sport – by either the amateur athlete or the professional athlete – can improve significantly after ART treatments.

Big names like Olympic gold-medalist Donovan Bailey, and hockey player Gary Roberts, and many others have benefited from ART and its ability to improve performance.

ART allows the body to perform at its most efficient level by restoring proper soft-tissue function and movement. Short, restricted structures are weak structures. The removal of these restrictions results in an almost immediate increase in strength. In addition, patients frequently experience improved reaction times due to improved muscular and nervous function.

For example, I worked with the ART Ironman team at the 2001 Ironman World Championships in Kona, Hawaii. As the last competitor crossed the finish line, I had a chance to talk to the race director about the results of the race. On that particular year, the heat was extreme, and the cross winds brutal. Despite these rough conditions, the race director was delighted to report that they had the highest percentage of finishers ever for this event. The race director attributed these remarkable results to the fact that over *one thousand ART treatments* were provided to athletes just prior to the event. These treatments resolved problems of tight tissues, restricted range-of-motions, and sometimes serious soft-tissue injuries, allowing the athletes to complete the event for which they had trained for so long.

It is not uncommon, after only a few ART sessions, to see a considerable improvement in the athlete's best personal performance. ART treatments return the body to a state that lets it perform the tasks that you ask of it – when you need it!

I have had an acute injury; how long must I wait before I can begin ART treatments?

For most cases, ART treatments can begin almost immediately after the occurrence of the acute injury. The sooner we start treating the injury, the faster and more complete the resolution.

It does not take long for tissue changes to occur after an injury. Just consider the following events that occur after an acute injury:

- First 24 to 72 hours – tissues become inflamed and swollen, with decreased circulation, and increased hypoxia (lack of oxygen) being delivered to the affected soft-tissues. During this stage use RICE to reduce the inflammation. See page 137 for details.

- Two days to two weeks later – the soft-tissue starts to become 'stringy' and the lesions within the soft-tissue become defined.

- Three weeks to three months later – the affected tissue becomes lumpy, with adhesions that are easily palpable.

- After three months – the adhesed tissues now have the consistency of leather.

Obviously, the sooner we can treat the restrictions, the better! So don't play the *wait-and-see* game!

Is there a difference between ART and other myo-fascial techniques?

Yes... ART is very different from any other soft-tissue technique, bodywork, massage, or other related therapies. ART is very specific in its treatment protocols, and is able to consistently achieve predictable results. For more information about ART and its relationship to other techniques, see the following:

- ART is not Massage Therapy! ---- page 16.
- ART is not Physiotherapy! ---- page 16.
- ART is not Chiropractic Care! ---- page 16.
- ART is not Surgery! ---- page 16.
- ART is not like other soft-tissue or myofascial techniques! ---- page 17.

What if my doctor recommends surgery?

There are situations when surgery is inevitable for the treatment of soft-tissue-related injury, but such situations are quite rare.

I am a strong believer in a multidisciplinary approach to health care. I am not against drugs, or surgery — when they are used appropriately. I strongly believe in the practice of '*responsible medicine*', where practitioners use the correct procedure at the correct time, and where alternatives to invasive procedures are encouraged and welcome.

As we have all heard, our current health care system is grossly overburdened. Doctors and other health care practitioners are generally elated when their patient's soft-tissue damage can be resolved without surgical intervention. And this is what ART can deliver.

Since ART is non-invasive and has no side effects, it is practical to try ART first to resolve any type of soft-tissue dysfunction. We commonly have patients who come to see us for a soft-tissue dysfunction while they are waiting for their scheduled surgery (which is often months later). When we are able to resolve their soft-tissue dysfunction, these excited patients generally report back to their physican for re-examination. The physican's tests often find that previously positive orthopedic and neurological tests are now showing negative. Even the gold-standard nerve condition tests show negative, indicating complete resolution of the initial problem. Given these kind of results, surgery is usually cancelled!

ART Practitioners

- How can I find out if my practitioner is certified in ART? ---- page 198.
- How do I find a certified ART practitioner in my area? ---- page 199.

How can I find out if my practitioner is certified in ART?

Be careful – there are many people who claim to practice Active Release Techniques, but who have not undergone the extensive training required.

Proficiency in ART takes time and training to develop. Training is hands-on. The right touch is the most difficult aspect to learn, and takes a strong commitment of time, effort, and resources.

The only individuals who are legally allowed to practice ART, have:

■ Completed and passed all three sections of ART (Spine, Upper Extremity, and Lower Extremity) and received their certification for Active Release Techniques.

■ Undergone rigorous training and testing with Dr. Michael Leahy by attending at least three, four-day workshops. Practitioners must pass both the written and practical examination with a greater than 90% proficiency.

■ Maintained their accreditation by passing a yearly evaluation and exam. This annual recertification process ensures that practitioners remain current with the latest changes and upgrades in the technique. Since ART is a rapidly evolving technique, it is critical that practitioners maintain their current skills and continually upgrade their methods with the new protocols that are generated each year.

Not everyone who claims to do ART has actually received the required training. Dr. Michael Leahy told me an amusing story that happened at an athletic event.

Apparently, Mike was working in a treatment area when an athlete asked if anyone there knew how to perform ART treatments. One doctor responded that he did, and began to work on the athlete.

Meanwhile, Mike (the developer of ART) stood by and watched the treatment take place. Unfortunately, none of the procedures that the doctor was performing was even remotely close to the ART protocols. Mike then asked the doctor, "*Is this Active Release Techniques that you are doing?*" The doctor responded, "*Yes, it is.*"

The doctor continued to treat the patient. After a while, Mike again asked, "*Are you sure this is ART?*" The doctor responded with, "*Yes, do you know any ART?*" To which Mike responded with a smile and said "*Actually, I invented it.*" To say the least, that doctor would have liked to have melted into the floor!

The bottom line is, make sure your practitioner is qualified to practice ART. Check out the website at www.activerelease.com to validate your practitioner's qualifications.

How do I find a certified ART practitioner in my area?

Active Release Techniques maintains a database of ART practitioners on their website. These practitioners are sorted by location, making it easy for you to find one close to your residence or work.

1. From your internet browser, navigate to www.activerelease.com.
2. Navigate to the section labelled 'Find a provider'.
3. Search for an ART provider by state, province, or zip code. Enter the distance you are willing to travel.
4. The search engine returns a list of providers within the area that you have selected.

About ART Treatments

- What are adhesions? ---- page 199.
- What is tissue translation? ---- page 200.
- What is nerve sliding or nerve flossing? ---- page 200.
- How long does an ART treatment take? ---- page 201.
- Are ART treatments painful? ---- page 201.

What are adhesions?

Our bodies contain special protein structures called *fascia* (a type of connective tissue). Fascial tissue interconnects and binds all the soft-tissue components of your body, and acts as a flexible skeleton. When this tissue is healthy, it is smooth and slippery, allowing the muscles, nerves, blood vessels, and organs to move freely and function properly.

Adhesions attach to muscles, ligaments, tendons, and nerves, decreasing their ability to work properly. A common sign of an adhesion causing compression on a nerve is an abnormal sensation of numbness, tingling, or pain.

To understand the impact of adhesions, imagine that you are holding a piece of scotch tape; the smooth side is healthy fascia, the sticky side is scar tissue or unhealthy fascia. Try rubbing both sides of the tape along your skin. The smooth side slips easily across your skin. The sticky side drags across your skin. The drag that you feel, the 'pulling' sensation, is similar to how an adhesion affects the smooth functioning of your body.

What is tissue translation?

Every motion you makes requires the movement or sliding of soft-tissue layers, nerves, and circulatory structures over each other, sometimes in the same direction, sometimes in opposing directions. This free, and uninhibited, sliding motion is critical to the proper functioning of these soft-tissues, and allows for effective biomechanics when carrying out any action.

In this book, we often speak about the importance of restoring tissue translation or motion to restricted soft-tissue. Restricted or adhesed tissues prevent this free sliding motion between layers of soft-tissue. These restrictions prevent the muscles and tissues from performing their required tasks, and cause the body to alter its biomechanics to a less than optimal state. By applying ART protocols to release these restrictions, we can restore the free translation of these soft-tissue structures, and thereby allow the body to function in a biomechanically correct manner.

What is nerve sliding or nerve flossing?

Every motion you makes requires the movement or sliding of tissue layers, nerves, and circulatory structures over each other. Most people do not think of nerves as structures that *move* within the body – but it is important to recognize that this movement does occur, and that it is required for the normal functioning of a nerve.

The term '*nerve sliding*' describes the action of the nerve sliding or moving between layers of muscle and connective tissue.

The nerves in your body are only loosely attached to the surrounding structures with connective tissue. In their normal, unrestricted state, all nerves have a considerable amount of mobility.

The ability of a nerve to function can be greatly altered and reduced when its *mobility is restricted*. This can happen when the surrounding structures around the nerve become injured, inflamed, or compressed. These stresses eventually lead to the formation of restrictive scar tissue that can encase and bind a nerve, preventing nerve sliding, and leading to dysfunctions such as numbness, tingling, and an inability to carry out physical tasks.

Nerve flossing refers to techniques that restore the relative motion between a nerve and its surrounding tissue. Many of the concepts of nerve flossing are integrated into the ART protocols that the practitioners use. In addition, many of the exercises in this book are designed to promote this relative translation between nerves and surrounding soft-tissue. By doing these exercises, you can reduce inflammation, reduce scar tissue formation, and help to restore mobility.

How long does an ART treatment take?

The initial consultation, history, examination, and treatment will usually require 30 minutes to one hour. Subsequent treatments take ten to fifteen minutes *per area* of the body being treated.

Are ART treatments painful?

The first one or two treatments can be somewhat uncomfortable depending on the severity of the condition and the patient's level of pain tolerance. The uncomfortable treatment phases occur during the movement stages as the scar tissue or adhesions 'break up'. This discomfort is temporary and subsides almost immediately after the treatment.

It is common to feel a duplication of your pain symptoms during the treatment (a good indication that the problem has been identified).

Post-Treatment

- What should I do directly after a treatment? ---- page 202.
- How long before I start seeing results with ART? ---- page 202.
- What are the chances of the injury reoccurring after ART treatments? ---- page 203.
- Why will exercises that did not work before, become effective after ART treatments? ---- page 203.
- Can I benefit from ART even after treatments by other doctors and specialists? ---- page 204.

What should I do directly after a treatment?

Remain active after an ART treatment. ART procedures produce structural changes in your body, and you need to *dial in those changes* by staying physically active. That is why, immediately after working on a patient, I will have them go for a walk, run, or do some activity that is related to their chief area of complaint.

How long before I start seeing results with ART?

Unlike most therapies, ART does not require extended periods of rest before you notice results. You can usually see significant improvements to the affected area after only two or three sessions.

In most cases, patients experience positive identifiable results almost immediately after the first treatment. These positive changes may manifest as increased range of motion, decreased pain, increased muscle strength, or decreased numbness and tingling. However, only 8% of patients get better after just the first treatment. Typically, 90% of patients find that their condition has resolved after 6 to 8 treatments.

What are the chances of the injury reoccurring after ART treatments?

Usually, ART-derived changes are permanent and long-lasting, but ultimately the answer depends upon the degree of patient compliance with post-care recommendations.

'If you keep doing what you're doing, you keep getting what you're getting'.

This is especially true for those suffering from repetitive strain injuries or cumulative trauma injuries. So...keep the following points in mind:

- Repetition of the injury-causing behavior or activities *will* cause the problem to reoccur. So, change this behavior to prevent reoccurrence of the injury.

- Follow the recommendations for modification of lifestyle and activity that are provided by your practitioner. These typically should include stretching, strengthening, balance, and cardiovascular exercises.

The likelihood of the condition reoccurring is very low when the patient implements the lifestyle modification recommendations and follows through with the prescribed exercises and stretches. For example, Dr. Leahy reported a reoccurrence rate of only 4% in his Carpal Tunnel study. Of these, half (2%) had *not* followed through with their exercises.

Why will exercises that did not work before, become effective after ART treatments?

Strengthening and stretching exercises are only effective if they are executed *after* the adhesions within the soft-tissue have been released. Attempts to strengthen muscles bound by adhesions often cause the structure to become more restricted, which in turn causes additional tension within the soft-tissue.

In addition to the strengthening and stretching aspects, balance and cardiovascular exercises continue to be key components for correcting the problem so that the RSI does not return.

Can I benefit from ART even after treatments by other doctors and specialists?

Only a provider experienced and trained in Active Release Techniques can determine if you might benefit from this treatment. Many of the cases that we see in our office are patients who have undergone unsuccessful treatments with other health care providers.

Most of these patients are happily surprised when they experience substantial improvements in their condition after just one or two treatments.

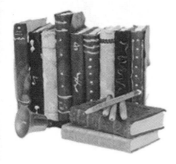

Glossary

The definitions in this glossary are provided from a soft-tissue/biomechanics perspective, and are oriented towards providing the general public with a better understanding of some of the technical terms that are used in this book. For more technical definitions, please refer to medical glossaries, many of which are available online on the world-wide web.

Achilles Tendonitis

A term used to describe an inflammation of the *paratenon* – a sheath surrounding the Achilles tendon. Achilles Tendonitis is often caused by overuse or repetitive strain and commonly occurs in triathletes and runners. See Injuries to the Achilles Tendon --- page 109 for more information.

adhesions

Normally, soft-tissue structures are often joined together by tough adhesive fibers. These are stable, strong structures. When adhesions form abnormally due to injuries, they can cause restrictions in movements and lead to further soft-tissue injuries.

amplitude

From a human biomechanics perspective, amplitude is a measurement of the degree of motion. For example, with RSI, the smaller the amplitude, the greater the degree of injury.

antagonists

Muscles whose actions oppose or counteract that of another set of muscles. For example, the triceps are the antagonists of the biceps.

anti-inflammatory

Any medication that can decrease inflammation or swelling within soft tissues.

biochemical

The biological and chemical changes that take place within the human body in response to environmental and physical changes.

biomechanical analysis - human

The study and evaluation of human motion with the goal of understanding how structures within the body affect each other. The study of biomechanics uses the principles of physics and mechanical engineering to find solutions to physical problems.

bursa

A bursa is a fibrous sac lined with synovial membrane and containing a small quantity of synovial fluid (joint fluid). Bursas function to facilitate fluid movement. Bursas act as a pad between tendons, bones, skin, and muscles.

bursitis

The inflammation of a bursa.

carpal tunnel syndrome

Carpal Tunnel Syndrome is traditionally described as a compression of the median nerve at the wrist. This compression can result in feelings of numbness, tingling, weakness, or muscle atrophy in the hand and fingers.

cartilage

Cartilage is the body's natural shock absorber, and enables your joints to support your weight when you bend, stretch, walk and run. There are different types of cartilage in the body:

- Articular cartilage covers the surfaces of your joints and is sometimes called hyaline cartilage.
- Fibrocartilage is found around your knees and spine.

cauda equina

A bundle of spinal nerve roots that arise from the termination points of the spinal cord. The cauda equina makes up the root of all the spinal nerves that originate below the first lumbar vertebrae.

circulatory system

The circulatory system is responsible for the transport of blood, oxygen, and nutrients to all the cells of your body. Restrictions which inhibit the flow of blood have an immediate impact upon soft-tissue function.

clavicle

Also known as the collarbone, to which the muscles of the neck and shoulder attach.

cortisone (corticosteroids)

Cortisone drugs are very powerful anti-inflammatory agents that are used to reduce inflammation and suppress activity of the immune system. They are the synthetic analogs of the natural cortisone that is produced by the body.

CTD - Cumulative Trauma Disorder

Another name for Repetitive Strain Injury (RSI).

CTS - Carpel Tunnel Syndrome

Another name for Repetitive Strain Injury (RSI).

diagnosis

The process by which a practitioner can determine the nature of a disease or dysfunction. The conclusion of this process is know as a diagnosis.

dorsiflexion

To bend the foot upwards.

edema

Describes the presence of an abnormally large amount of fluid in the intercellular tissue spaces of the body. Edema often occurs with soft-tissue injuries that have caused inflammation and which have reduced circulation to the affected tissues.

ergonomics

The study of human factors involved in the design and operation of machines, as well as the study of the physical environment in which people have to work and live.

eversion

The inward rolling of the foot during gait.

fascia

The flat layers of fibrous tissue that separate different layers of soft-tissue. Fascia should be smooth and slippery to allow easy translation of soft-tissue layers over each other. Adhesions binding these tissue layers cause fascia to become rough, causing restricted motions, increased friction, and the exacerbation of the Cumulative Injury Cycle.

femur

A large bone in the thigh that connects to and articulates with the pelvis above, and the knee below.

fulcrum

A point in the body against which a structure can act as a lever, or against which it can turn, lift or move the body.

hypoxia

A condition where oxygen supply to tissues is reduced to below optimal levels. Hypoxia frequently occurs when tissues are inflamed or restricted.

immobilization

The act of rendering all or part of the body immobile, whether accidentally or deliberately.

impingement (Impingement Syndrome)

Impingement syndrome describes a condition where there is a mechanical obstruction (impingement) between soft-tissue structures.

incontinence

The inability to control excretory functions, such as defecation (faecal incontinence) or urination (urinary incontinence).

inversion

The outward rolling of the foot during gait.

kinetic chain

All the neurological and soft-tissue structures that are associated with, or whose actions affect, another structure in the body. Every muscle, ligament, tendon, nerve and fascia has its own unique chain of structures that affect its function. Restrictions in the structures of the kinetic chain can have a cascading effect on other structures and upon general body biomechanics.

knee cap

Also known as the patella. The knee cap is a common site of repetitive stress injuries. See Bones of the Knee --- page 127 for more information.

lateral

Describes a structure lying on the outer side of body or away from the midline of the body.

ligaments

Bands of fibrous tissue that connect bones and cartilage, and serve to support and strengthen joints. See Ligaments of the Knee --- page 127 for more information.

medial

Describes structures that lie towards the center of the body.

meniscus

A circular-shaped cartilage in your knee that acts as a shock absorber – helping to spread out the weight that is transferred (during gait) from the femur to the tibia. See Meniscus --- page 128 for more information.

MRI

Magnetic Resonance Imaging – used to obtain images of soft-tissue structures. See MRI (Magnetic resonance imaging) --- page 132 and The value of MRI --- page 175 for more information.

mRNA

This is a type of RNA that is found in all cells. mRNA is a copy of a single protein-coding gene in your genome and acts as a template for protein synthesis. Each mRNA provided a unique template for generating a specific protein structure.

Anything which interferes with mRNA production or function will directly affect your body's ability to build muscle, and repair damaged cell walls. It will also cause an increase in fibroblast cells, which help to lay down scar tissue, forming adhesions. See The Cumulative Injury Cycle --- page 12 for more information about how RSIs affect mRNA production.

myofascial tissues

Tissues that are part of, or that are related to, the fascia that surrounds and separates layers of muscle.

nerve flossing

Nerve flossing refers to techniques that restore the relative motion between a nerve and its surrounding tissue. Nerve flossing can be accomplished through ART protocols or by specific exercises. See What is nerve sliding or nerve flossing? --- page 200 for more details.

nerve sliding

Describes the normal sliding or movement of nerves between layers of muscle and connective tissue. See What is nerve sliding or nerve flossing? --- page 200 for more details.

neuromuscular

Pertaining to both muscles and nerves.

NSAIDs

Non-steroidal anti-inflammatory drugs, that are used to temporarily relieve pain, swelling, and inflammation.

Non-steroidal anti-inflammatory drugs can cause a number of side effects, some of which may be very serious. These side effects are more likely when the drugs are taken in large doses or for a long time or when two or more non-steroidal anti-inflammatory drugs are taken together.

osteoporosis

A reduction in the amount of bone mass. Reduced bone mass leads to fractures after even minimal trauma, and is a leading cause of physical dysfunction in North America.

paratenon

A connective sheath that surrounds the Achilles tendon. See Achilles Tendonitis/ Paratenonitis --- page 112 for more details.

patella

The technical term for the knee cap. The patella is a common site of repetitive strain injuries. See Bones of the Knee --- page 127 for more details.

peripheral nerves

The peripheral nerves are responsible for relaying information from your central nervous system (brain and spinal cord) to muscles and other organs. When entrapped by restrictions, injury, or trauma, patients may experience loss of function, tingling, or pain in their extremities.

plantar fascia

The plantar fascia is a thin band of fibrous tissue that runs from the calcaneus (heel bone) to the base of the toes.

plantar fasciitis

Plantar Fasciitis is most often described as an inflammation of the plantar aponeurosis or plantar fascia. See Plantar Fasciitis --- page 95 for more information.

plantar flexion

The act of pointing your toe.

pronated

The inward rolling of the foot or hand. If your wrist is in a pronated position your palm would be face down.

proprioception

Describes the body's ability to react appropriately (through balance and touch) to external forces. Tissue restrictions cause changes in the body's biomechanics which in turn affects your sense of balance.

After ART treatments have removed restrictions that have altered your normal biomechanics, exercises in each chapter of this book can help you to restore your sense of proprioception.

pseudo

False or mimicked symptoms of a more commonly known dysfunction. See Why ART is so Successful --- page 40 for more information.

quadriceps

A group of four muscles at the front of your thigh: rectus femoris, vastus lateralis, vastus intermedius, and vastus medialis. These muscles act as your secondary hip flexors. Your primary hip flexors are your psoas and iliacus muscles.

RNA

An acronym for ribonucleic acid. RNA acts as an intermediary, transcribing the DNA to generate a template that is used for the creation of proteins.

rotator cuff

The rotator cuff is a tendon formed by four distinct muscles – subscapularis, infraspinatus, teres minor, and supraspinatus. These muscles stabilize the head of the humerus within the shoulder joint. See Rotator Cuff Muscles --- page 76 for more information.

RSI

The acronym for Repetitive Strain Injury. See chapters one and two for more information about RSIs.

scapula

The technical term for shoulder blade. See Scapula or Shoulder Blade --- page 77 for more information.

sequestered disc

When material from a spinal disc completely separates from the parent disc and floats independently in the spinal channel. See Disc Herniation, Protrusion, Prolapse, & Extrusion --- page 167 for more information.

shin bone

The common term for the tibia. This large bone lies between the knee and foot and supports 70% of the body's weight.

soft-tissues

Soft-tissues refers to muscles, ligaments, tendons, nerves, fascia, and circulatory and lymphatic structures.

supinating

A rolling motion to the outside edge of the foot during a step. If you are supinating your wrist, your palm would end face-up.

symptomatic relief

Treatments which only treat the *symptoms* rather than the *cause* of injury. See The Traditional Perspective --- page 79 for more information.

tendonitis

Inflammation of the tendons.

tendons

Tendons are extremely strong cords of connective tissue that connect muscle to bone, and are the termination point of muscles.

tibia

The technical term for shin bone. This large bone lies between the knee and foot and supports 70% of the body's weight.

translation of soft-tissues

The term *translation* (as used in this book) refers to the restoration of relative motion between adjacent soft-tissue layers.

Every motion you make requires the movement or sliding of soft-tissue layers, nerves, and circulatory structures over each other – sometimes in the same direction, sometimes in opposing directions. This free and uninhibited sliding motion is critical to the proper functioning of these soft-tissues, and allows for effective biomechanics when carrying out any action. See *What is tissue translation? --- page 200* for more information.

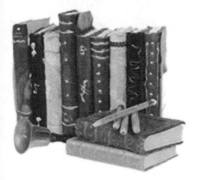

Index

B

L

M

R

repetitive strain injuries
    See RSI

restrictions
    removing with ART 18

rotator cuff
    about 76, 80
    ART treatments 81
    case history 85
    definition of 211
    impingements 80
    muscles of 76

RSI
    about 1, 2
    causes of 2, 8
    common solutions 1
    Cumulative Injury Cycle 12
    economics of 5
    Law of Repetitive Motion 10, 43
    occupations affected 4
    prevalence of 4, 33
    solutions for 1, 6
    statistics 5
    symptoms of 7, 8
    types of 2, 9
    what it is? 2

Runner's Knee
    see ITBS

S

scapula
    about 77
    definition of 211
    exercises 89

sciatica
    back pain 170
    patient's story 182

sequestered disc
    definition of 211

shoulder
    about 75
    bones 75, 77
    exercises 88–94
    function of 74
    injuries 73
    muscles 75, 76, 77, 78
    rotator cuff 76
    scapula 77
    structures 75, 76, 77, 78

shoulder injuries
    ART treatments 81, 84
    case history 85
    causes of 74, 80
    exercises 88–94
    frozen shoulder 82
    impingements 80
    patients' story 85
    rotator cuff 80, 85
    sufferers 74
    symptoms of 9, 73
    tendonitis 80
    traditional treatments 79
    treatment problems 79

soft tissues
    ART treatments for 18
    Cumulative Injury Cycle 12
    definition of 211
    removing restrictions 18

splinting 48
    Carpal Tunnel Syndrome 34, 42
    Plantar Fasciitis 103

steroids
    carpal tunnel syndrome 48
    definition of 207
    shoulder injuries 79
    side-effects of 48, 79

surgery 16
    back pain 156
    Carpal Tunnel Syndrome 35, 49
    compared to ART 16
    costs of 135
    functional resolution criteria 39
    knee injuries 126, 136
    side-effects of 42, 49
    statistics 33, 135
    value of 177